THE STRESS EFFECT

EFFECT

Discover the Connection Between Stress
and Illness and Reclaim Your Health

RICHARD WEINSTEIN, D.C.

AVERY
a member of Penguin Group (USA) Inc.
New York

AVERY

a member of
Penguin Group (USA) Inc.
375 Hudson Street
New York, NY 10014
www.penguin.com

Library of Congress Cataloging-in-Publication Data

Weinstein, Richard (Richard A.)
The stress effect : discover the connection between stress and illness
and reclaim your health / Richard Weinstein.
p.   cm.
Includes bibliographical references and index.
ISBN 1-58333-181-6
1. Medicine, Psychosomatic.   2. Stress (Psychology).   3. Stress (Psychology—Health
aspects).   4. Stress management—Health aspects.   I. Title.
RC49.W395   2004   2003057735
616.08—dc22

Printed in the United States of America
1   3   5   7   9   10   8   6   4   2

Book design by Stephanie Huntwork

For Lois, my dearest friend, my beloved wife,
and the finest person I have ever known

ACKNOWLEDGMENTS

This book is the result of more than two decades of clinical experience and a continuous learning process in keeping up with research on hormonal function and imbalances, and how to resolve them. There are two groups of wonderful people to thank in making this book a reality: those who mentored me to become a better doctor and taught me the pieces of the hormone physiological puzzle, and those who enabled me to write and publish this book.

First and foremost, my heartfelt thanks to Harry O. Eidenier, Jr., Ph.D., who gave me the initial inkling of how to make sense of the incredible complexities of the human hormone system, and who has generously lent his time, support, and profound wisdom for this project. My thanks to David R. Seaman, D.C., who is a visionary regarding the destructive impact of inflammation on human health, and to Dan Murphy, D.C., who is a brilliant teacher of neurology and the dynamics of joint function. Anyone who either studies or writes about the subject of stress owes an enormous debt of gratitude to Robert M. Sapolsky, Ph.D., the Stanford University researcher who, by all standards, is a modern-day genius of human stress physiology, and who is also a wonderful and often hilarious writer, and a truly great human being.

A big hug and thanks to Dario Ciriello, who did the initial editing of my book, who kept me focused and on track, and who always believed in the value of this project. Writing a book is one thing, but getting it published is a completely different process, and without the invaluable help of my literary agent, Sandra Bond, you would not be holding this book in your hands. Sandra is every writer's dream come true, an agent who meticulously guided this book to its completion, and I feel truly blessed to have her as my agent. My sincere thanks to Dara Stewart, my editor at Avery, for her sound advice and generous help in guiding this book through the publishing process. I would also like to thank my sister, Gerrie Nachman, for introducing me to authors Lois Machamie and Patricia Ensworth, who graciously shared their experiences of the world of writing and publishing with me, and prepared me for the ups and downs of being a writer. To Dick Bruso, another hug and thanks for his excellent advice and help in showing me the best approach to getting this book out to the reading public.

Last, writing a book is a very time-consuming enterprise, and it can be a challenge if you already have a full-time job, as I do with my practice. None of this would have been possible without the support of my wife, Lois, and her tireless efforts to pick up the slack in managing my office and our home while I sat at the computer, writing. Clearly, I have a lot of lawns to mow and dishes to wash to make up for all of this, and I am forever grateful for her loving support.

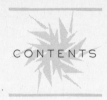

CONTENTS

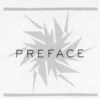

This book will enable you to look at stress from a totally new perspective and to understand that stress isn't always a matter of how you psychologically respond to the circumstances in your life, but a matter of how stress hormones can be coursing through your body on a daily basis in response to internal inflammation. Most books about stress want to convince us that stress and the symptoms related to it are due to the hectic, multitasking lives we lead, and allow us to assume that it is natural to feel emotionally overwhelmed. As a result, we have been led to believe that if we just change our attitudes, meditate, exercise, and/or do yoga for an hour or so every day, we will no longer be stressed-out. Exactly how we are supposed to find the time to fit all of this into what is presumed to be our busy, stressful lives never seems to be a concern in these books.

The idea that stress is completely psychological is not scientifically accurate, and it ignores the significant role of internal inflammation as a cause of imbalance in our stress-hormone levels. You see, the hormone that our body secretes in times of stress is the same hormone it uses to resolve inflammation. This hormone, called *cortisol,* is secreted by our adrenal glands. The irony in this is that taking anti-inflammatory medications—your average, everyday painkillers—causes intestinal-tract inflammation by inhibiting the enzymes necessary for the intestinal tract to replenish and repair itself, and eventually can lead to chronic inflammation. The overuse of antibiotics can also cause intestinal-tract damage, and the average, imbalanced American diet of processed foods, fast foods, caffeine, and alcohol also contributes to intestinal-tract inflammation as well as systemic inflammation in our bodies.

In this book, we are going to look at *all* of the components of stress, and we are going to use the holistic model called the *triangle of health* to resolve stress and its effects. The three components of the triangle are *structural* integrity, *chemical* integrity, and *psychological* integrity, and when all three components are well balanced, we have optimal health. The structural component refers to the health of the body's tissues and the body's alignment; the chemical component refers to diet and hormonal balance; and the psychological component refers to our thoughts and emotional well-being.

Within months of starting my private chiropractic practice twenty-five years ago, it became apparent to me that stress was a major factor in human health disorders. I became fascinated by the way stress affected people so very differently and how there seemed to be some mysterious, hidden factor behind its effects. I would treat patients who didn't seem to have that many problems in their lives (not counting whatever pain syndrome they were experiencing) but who felt that they were totally overwhelmed and stressed-out. They were depressed; not sleeping well; craving sugar, salt, and caffeine; and having mood swings throughout the day. Then there would be other patients whose personal lives appeared to be a virtual shipwreck who, other than suffering the discomfort of a backache or neck pain, were doing fine.

Seeing these types of cases over and over again intrigued me and caused me to look at and study stress from a perspective that perhaps it isn't as emotionally based as it appears on the surface. I began to consider the possibility that maybe much of what I was seeing in these patients who felt so stressed-out was due to *chemical* or *structural* imbalances that were causing a hypersensitive response to the normal challenges of daily life.

Fortunately, years of scientific research regarding stress has concluded that cortisol is a major culprit as the *chemical* factor behind all of this suffering. Cortisol imbalances have been scientifically linked to obesity, diabetes, depression, heart disease, insomnia, autoimmune diseases like chronic fatigue syndrome, thyroid disorders, ulcers, irritable bowel syndrome, and even osteoporosis. While it is true that cortisol is the hormone that is secreted when we are confronted with life-threatening "fight-or-flight" stress and also when we are emotionally distressed, might there still be a *structural* trigger that causes cortisol secretion? As a classic case of which came first, the chicken or the egg, might it not be possible that a *structural* trigger elevates your cortisol levels first, and then you feel that circumstances in your life are more stressful that they would be if your cortisol levels were normal? Well, yes, there is! It's inflammation.

As it turns out, cortisol is also the body's natural anti-inflammatory chemical, and any time there is inflammation, there will be cortisol secretion in response to it. The *structural* trigger is inflammation, and, again, most of the time it occurs in the intestinal tract as a result of taking anti-inflammatory medications and/or antibiotics and having a diet that promotes inflammation.

This book is designed to help you understand the three components of stress and will serve as a guide to show you how to correct imbalances in all three of these components and regain your health.

I am inviting you to take a journey with me and see stress in a completely different light. Your experience will likely be similar to that of a person who doesn't realize how bad his vision is until he puts on a pair of corrective eyeglasses. If your cortisol levels are imbalanced, it can be very difficult to understand that your feelings of being overwhelmed, anxious, depressed, frightened, or worried most of the time are *not* natural. Your symptoms of fatigue, inability to sleep, food cravings, and weight gain are also *not* natural, but they can be resolved once you read this book and find out what the true cause of these symptoms is.

THE STRESS EFFECT

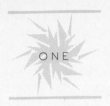

THE BEGINNING
OF THE JOURNEY

A Chiropractor's Odyssey with Stress

My interest in the adrenal glands, cortisol levels, the human response to stress, inflammation, and the effects of cortisol on health was a gift from my patients. Certainly, endocrine or hormonal systems are studied as part of the anatomy and physiology courses that are taught in chiropractic colleges, but I can't say that at the time I found them all that intriguing or particularly relevant to what I thought I would be doing as a practicing chiropractor.

In the chiropractic college curriculum, there is a great emphasis on the philosophy of chiropractic, including the triangle of health. In this paradigm, the three components of health are structural integrity, chemical integrity, and psychological integrity. Structural integrity refers to spinal and joint alignment, muscle tone, ligament stability and flexibility, and the physical status of all of the body's tissues and organs. Chemical integrity involves our diets and the foods, liquids, drugs, and other chemicals we put into our bodies. It also includes the balance of our hormones and neurotransmitters, which control the metabolic functions of both body and mind. The third part of the triangle is the psychological aspect. It would probably be impossible to buy a self-help book or tape that doesn't emphasize the importance of positive thinking or the concept that you are what you think. Whereas as recently as fifteen years ago the mind/body connection was laughed at by practitioners of traditional medicine, doctors such as Andrew Weil and Deepak Chopra have brought it into the mainstream of public consciousness.

UNDERSTANDING THE EFFECTS OF STRESS

While all of the aspects of the triangle of health are addressed in chiropractic college, there is no doubt that the emphasis is placed on the structural part, as it is the mission and purpose of chiropractic care to ensure the structural integrity of the body by adjusting or aligning the spinal and peripheral joints. So, with a somewhat limited background in chemical integrity, my real journey deep into the "land of the adrenals" began in my first year of practice with a twenty-eight-year-old male patient with multiple joint complaints. It seemed like just about everything hurt: his neck, his lower back, his knees, his elbows, and even his ankles. He was able to function, but the pain was seriously limiting the quality of his life.

After taking a complete history and performing a thorough examination, I initiated a treatment program that consisted of adjusting the painful joints, along with applying cold compresses and performing corrective exercises at home. He responded very well, and the intensity and frequency of his pain progressively diminished to the point where, after one month of care, he was stable and about to be released from further treatment.

Then one day he came to my office for what I thought would be his last follow-up visit, and nearly all of his symptoms had returned. There was no new injury or accident to account for his pain, and I tried various avenues of questioning in an effort to determine what had caused this sudden recurrence of his symptoms. We went through everything from whether he had been lifting, gardening, or house cleaning; had he slept in a poor position, and on and on, with absolutely no clue as to what could be the cause of his recurring pain.

At a loss for any reasonable explanation for a structural cause of his pain, I took a shot at the psychological component and asked if he had encountered any new or unusually stressful situations. It didn't take but a few seconds before he launched into a diatribe about how his little momma from Miami had been visiting for the past two weeks, and she was driving him crazy!

With no disrespect to my own mother, let's just say I had an inkling of, and considerable empathy for, the stress he was experiencing. It gave me my first graphic clinical insight into how dramatic an effect stress can have on structural alignment and pain. It taught me from then on to always consider a patient's stress profile in determining both the cause and treatment of his problems. With regard to this young man, I gave him an adrenal glandular supplement to nutritionally support his adrenal glands, and within a few weeks he was fine again.

As the years went by, I continued to hone my skills by attending a wide variety of seminars that addressed the advances in research regarding neurology, nutrition, joint biomechanics, muscle balancing, and craniosacral therapy. I felt I had a good grasp on how to treat my patients effectively and help them with their problems. Everything was going along just fine, and then Marilyn entered my office and forever changed my world.

MARILYN

I had been in practice for sixteen years when Marilyn came in as a new patient and presented a history unlike anything I had ever encountered. About a year before she came to see me, she had been a long-distance runner, averaging forty miles a week, and was employed full-time in a highly responsible and stressful position in law enforcement.

Her odyssey began when she developed a persistent burning pain in her esophagus. She went for a medical checkup, and all of her tests proved negative for disease. As her condition worsened, further testing revealed blood in her stools and a lowered red-blood-cell count. She began to experience extreme fatigue and weakness, along with multiple joint pains, and she was hospitalized to undergo more tests.

Marilyn's condition continued to worsen, with pain in her knees, elbows, hands, and pelvis; headaches; dizziness; chest pain; difficulty breathing; and insomnia. Her lungs had weakened to the point that, by the time she entered my office, she became exhausted after just fifteen minutes of talking, and her overall physical condition had declined so dramatically that she could only walk two blocks before becoming too fatigued to go any farther.

As her symptoms progressed, she sought help from a gastrointestinal specialist, a pulmonary specialist, an endocrinologist (hormone specialist), and Stanford University Hospital. Yet here she was in my office, referred by her brother, with her condition showing no signs of improvement and with no end in sight.

Where to begin was no problem for me, for as a chiropractor, it was obvious that her condition had been approached medically from just about every angle and that the only treatments she had yet to receive were spinal adjustments and acupuncture. So I adjusted her spine and the other affected joints, performed craniosacral therapy, gave her corrective exercises, advised her to use cold compresses at home, and placed her on an oral adrenal-gland supplement.

Marilyn returned for her second visit two days later, and it appeared as if a miracle had occurred. She was breathing better and could walk longer distances; the burning pain in her esophagus was gone, and her back and joint pain was greatly reduced. With each subsequent visit, her condition got progressively better, and I figured that I was next in line for the Nobel Prize.

Then Marilyn introduced me to the phenomenon of adrenal rebound. One month after beginning treatment with me, during which all of her symptoms had improved, the bottom fell out. Marilyn began to have trouble sleeping again, and her fatigue and joint pain were returning. I had no clue as to what would make this happen, since no other factors in her life had changed, and the treatment program hadn't been altered.

What I couldn't have known at the time, because there just wasn't much research available, was that the adrenal glands have a nasty tendency to "rebound," which means that they can initially respond well to the administration of an adrenal-gland-extract supplement, but if the *cause* of the cortisol imbalance is not addressed, they will "rebound," restoring the imbalance.

About this time, Marilyn also consulted with a medical doctor who had begun specializing in female hormonal disorders. Dr. Kathryn Morris introduced both of us to salivary hormonal testing, and Marilyn's test revealed that her adrenal glands were in a maladaptive phase in which her cortisol levels were elevated and her DHEA (another adrenal hormone) levels were depressed. So while I was initially able to support her adrenal glands with supplements, I hadn't raised or balanced the DHEA part of the equation. Dr. Morris prescribed DHEA for Marilyn in progressively increasing doses.

Marilyn improved immediately when she began taking the DHEA, and all of her symptoms once more began to settle down. However, this again proved to be short lived. The problem, unbeknownst to all of us, was that we still had not discovered the *cause* of her adrenal-gland malfunction.

Dr. Morris and I—and most of all Marilyn—persevered and kept trying different supplements and approaches. We ran the gamut from more adrenal extracts to vitamin-B_{12} injections, increasing dietary essential fatty acids, thyroid testing, and subsequent thyroid medication. It was a long, long road to recovery, and every aspect of hormonal balancing had to be addressed.

It was also a dramatic illustration of just how many things can go wrong hormonally, how intricately the organs that make up the hormonal system are interconnected, and what a very delicate balance the hormonal system must maintain. While Marilyn's symptom complex had no definitive medical name back then, today she would be diagnosed with both chronic fatigue syndrome and fibromyalgia.

The happy ending to this story is that Marilyn did eventually fully recover. Through the relentless rebalancing of her hormones and the process of time, her body was able to heal, and she is now able to run, lift weights, and lead a functionally normal life. She still requires DHEA and adrenal supplementation to keep her adrenal glands balanced, but she has her life back.

Marilyn's case took a particularly long time to resolve because of the severity of her condition and the fact that at the time, so little was known about these kinds of problems. This, unfortunately, led to a lot of trial and error as we were learning how to effect a positive change. In addition, nobody at that time realized that intestinal-tract inflammation, which can be caused by psychological stress, anti-inflammatory medications, caffeine, alcohol, or any combination of these factors, could trigger the whole cascade of adrenal-gland imbalance. Besides being the hormone that handles stress, cortisol is also the body's anti-inflammatory hormone. Much like the adage "Where there's smoke, there's fire," where there is inflammation, there will be elevated levels of cortisol.

Had I known then what I know now, I would have suspected that there was intestinal inflammation, based on the fact that one of her initial symptoms was the burning sensation in her esophagus and the eventual blood in her stools. What caused the intestinal-tract problem was not anti-inflammatory medications, antibiotics, or a poor diet, but the chronic emotional stress of her job, for which she ultimately received a total disability exemption. Fortunately, by learning from our experiences and better research, these hormonal problems are now easier to resolve.

While it was unfortunate for Marilyn that her case was exceptionally complicated, in the long run it was of great benefit to me. Attempting to solve her health problems was a very humbling experience because each time she seemed to be on the verge of recovery, some other aspect of her hormonal system would go awry. This inspired me to learn as much as I could about the intricacies of the endocrine system so that I could become more proficient in treating hormone imbalances and less frustrated when patients did not respond as I thought they should.

The Road to Enlightenment

After reading extensively about the endocrine system in order to fully grasp how the hormone system works and how the different hormones affect each other, I began to attend seminars given by Diagnos-Techs, the laboratory that analyzed Marilyn's salivary adrenal stress index test. I was amazed at the amount of scientific information these researchers had available. The seminars were eye-opening experiences that put me firmly on the path of understanding the correlation between intestinal-tract inflammation and cortisol imbalances. The doctors teaching these seminars were very clear in stating all of the causes of adrenal-gland imbalances and in warning the doctors in the audience not to assume that all adrenal problems have their basis in psychological stress. They were also adamant in their belief that we would be wasting our time and our patients' money if we neglected to treat the *cause* of the adrenal imbalance as opposed to its symptoms. This advice certainly made me think of Marilyn's case.

It was in the Diagnos-Techs seminars I first learned about secretory IgA, an antibody that binds to specific antigens and harmful microorganisms to *prevent* their attachment to the intestinal-tract lining. Secretory IgA decreases with physical pain and mental stress, with inflammation caused by the prolonged use of nonsteroidal anti-inflammatory medications and/or antibiotics, with the dietary abuses of too much caffeine and alcohol, or with a combination of all of these factors, and as a result is unable to perform its protective function. An adrenal stress index test that reveals abnormally low levels of secretory IgA signals the doctor that the intestinal tract is inflamed and that, unless this condition is resolved, the cortisol levels will most certainly remain imbalanced.

After attending the Diagnos-Techs seminars, I had the good fortune to meet Dr. Harry O. Eidenier, Jr., who has a doctorate in chemistry and who is one of the smartest people I have ever had the pleasure to meet. Through the serendipitous wonder of mass mailing,

I received information about a series of seminars that Dr. Eidenier was giving. Called "Balancing Body Chemistry with Nutrition," they dealt with this very same subject of hormonal imbalances and the advances being made in treating them with nutritional supplements. Once again, the core issue of intestinal-tract inflammation as a precursor to hormone imbalance was a central theme, and the doctors in attendance were exhorted to think in terms of the potential physical causes of cortisol imbalances and not just psychological factors.

I learned about the final piece of the puzzle, systemic inflammation, in a seminar by Dr. David R. Seaman, a chiropractor who also has a master's degree in nutrition. Dr. Seaman was years ahead of medical research in his knowledge of the importance of diet in elevating inflammatory chemicals (prostaglandins) in the body to a level where they can cause pain and tissue damage.

So, after years of studying and attending seminars on the subject, correcting hormonal imbalances is now a routine part of my practice and something I expect to deal with in the normal course of my workday. Having had so much experience in this area, I find many cases easy to treat because I see similar patterns of symptoms so often.

THE FIRST SIGNS OF TROUBLE

When a new patient comes to my office, the first thing I do is sit down with him or her and inquire about the structural, chemical, and, if appropriate, the psychological components of that person's health. Because cortisol can affect nearly every system in our bodies, the list of symptoms associated with cortisol imbalance seems almost endless. The most common ones are cravings for salt, sugar, or carbohydrates; mood swings and irritability; fluctuation in energy levels throughout the day; and feeling that the daily demands of life are overwhelming.

One of the more important symptoms of cortisol imbalance I see on a regular basis is insomnia, which is often the first serious indicator of cortisol imbalance. Usually, falling asleep is not a problem, but by two or three o'clock in the morning, the patient is wide awake for thirty minutes or longer. This type of insomnia is a classic sign of cortisol imbalance because by nighttime, cortisol levels should be very low; if they are abnormally high, they will trigger a state of alertness that will cause this sleep pattern. Probably everyone has experienced this sleep pattern in his or her life when there is a particular worry or stressful situation to deal with, and if it only occurs very occasionally, it is not much of a concern. However, in my practice, I see patients who tell me that this is a consistent pattern that they have lived with for years, and for me, as a chiropractor, it has a special significance.

An obvious part of getting any patient well is the healing process, and with chiropractic care, the emphasis is on repairing and healing connective tissue, such as ligaments, tendons, and muscles, associated with the joints. It's great to be able to put a misaligned joint back into alignment and restore it to its normal range of motion and bio-mechanical capabilities, but if the connective tissues that hold it in alignment don't properly heal, the joint is likely to pop back out of alignment again.

The connective tissue of the body undergoes a daily repair process that occurs while we are sleeping. A consistent pattern of insomnia inhibits the ability of these tissues to heal, and the likelihood of achieving joint stability is greatly reduced. And not only is it the connective tissue of joints that are of concern, but once again it's also the intestinal-tract lining and other tissues of the body that are not repaired if we are not sleeping.

There are many types of adrenal and related hormone imbalances that I treat on a daily basis, and it is truly gratifying to be able to help people get well—not just better, not just symptom free, but completely well—and function in a state of true health. The success in resolving these cases lies in correlating the components of the triangle of health with the patient's individual symptoms and needs, and in making sure the structural, chemical, and psychological components are well balanced. Thank you, Marilyn, for all that you taught me.

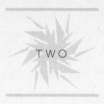

TWO

THE PARADOX
OF CORTISOL

The Hormone of Stress and Inflammation

Now it's time to meet our good friend cortisol, the primary hormone of stress and the body's anti-inflammatory chemical. If we are to make sense of the far-reaching effects of the human stress response and the far-reaching effects of inflammation on our bodies, then we are going to have to become acquainted with how the system works. Essentially, as with most systems in our bodies, the hormonal system is a negative feedback loop. This means that we produce specific chemicals to initiate specific reactions, and when they rise to a level of overabundance, the system triggers a mechanism to turn it off. This is similar to the relationship between the furnace and thermostat in your home. The thermostat is a temperature-sensitive switch: Set to seventy-two degrees, it will signal the furnace to turn on when the ambient temperature drops below this level. As the temperature rises beyond the desired setting, this again triggers the thermostat, causing it to shut down the furnace. In the human body, this delicate mechanism of balance is referred to as *homeostasis,* and it is largely regulated by the autonomic nervous system.

The Autonomic Nervous System: Pedal to the Metal or Putting on the Brakes

The underlying neurology that orchestrates the human stress response resides in the autonomic nervous system, which is divided into the sympathetic and parasympathetic branches. The autonomic nervous system oversees the neurological functions that we don't have to voluntarily control, such as breathing, digestion, blood pressure, blinking, and, for some politicians, thinking. It is important to note, however, that through techniques such as biofeedback, meditation, and psychoneuroimmunology, some of these functions can be consciously controlled.

The sympathetic branch of the autonomic nervous system is the one that gets things going and is activity oriented. You have sympathetic nerve endings in almost every organ, muscle, and blood vessel to facilitate its function. The adrenal glands also secrete the hormones epinephrine and norepinephrine to stimulate the sympathetic system in times of stress.

On the other end of the neurological spectrum is the parasympathetic branch, which puts the brakes on the system. It's great to be able to pump out hormones that will increase your heart rate, respiration, blood pressure, and muscle strength for exercise or for responding to physical danger, but you can't go on like that indefinitely without causing trouble. The parasympathetic system is the counterbalance to sympathetic activity that restores calm, promotes relaxation, and facilitates digestive functions, energy storage, and tissue repair and growth. It is the vast difference between these two branches that explains why your parents admonished you as a child not to go swimming until an hour after you had eaten lunch. You run the risk of life-threatening muscle cramping when you try to send your blood to your digestive tract and to skeletal muscles at the same time.

As the sympathetic system becomes engaged in the stress response, be it physiological or psychological, a whole cascade of hormonal events occurs. It is very important to point out that while this system was intended for physical stressors that endangered survival, it operates exactly the same way when the stress is psychological and not life threatening. Of course, if you are teaching your teenager to drive, then it's going to be both. As you might imagine, it all begins in your brain and specifically the limbic system and neocortex. The limbic system is the more emotional or feeling part, whereas the neocortex deals more with thinking. Both are located in the largest part of the brain, the cerebrum.

The Limbic System and the Awareness of Stress

The limbic system is composed of the hippocampus, the thalamus, the hypothalamus, the pituitary gland, and the amygdala. This is essentially a system of interconnected relay stations that converse with each other in microseconds. Simply put, the thalamus receives all incoming information and disperses it out to: (1) the hippocampus, which stores short-term and nonemotional fact-based memory; (2) the amygdala, which processes and stores emotional memory; and (3) the neocortex, or thinking part of the brain. After these three structures evaluate the stimulus coming from the thalamus and determine its importance, then the hypothalamus can get into the act by releasing hormones. If the stimulus is deemed stressful, the hypothalamus releases CRF (corticotrophin-releasing factor), which then goes to the pituitary gland. Now, I realize that this is getting a little complicated, and by now you may not really care if the hippocampus is in your brain or a place where aquatic African mammals attend college, but this will all become relevant when we see what happens to these structures when the stress response gets out of control.

The pituitary gland responds to the CRF by releasing ACTH (adrenocorticotropin hormone) into the bloodstream, where it signals the adrenal glands to release glucocorticoids, which we will hereafter refer to as cortisol. This chain of hormonal events can take a few minutes, so for an immediate stress response, epinephrine (adrenaline) is released from the sympathetic nerve endings throughout the body. Although over the years adrenaline has gained a bad reputation as the stress hormone, the body utilizes it only for the first two to five minutes of the stress response, after which it is cortisol that takes over and choreographs the rest of the stress response.

As with the thermostat-and-furnace feedback loop, upon initiation of the stress response, the hypothalamus releases CRF, and the pituitary gland releases ACTH, which causes the adrenal glands to secrete cortisol. Once the stress is resolved, the cortisol circulates back to the hypothalamus, and the system shuts down. With chronic or repetitive stress, however, the hypothalamus can become desensitized to cortisol and unable to stop the pituitary gland from signaling the adrenal glands to keep secreting cortisol. This is like the thermostat in your home malfunctioning and not knowing when it is hot enough and not being able to turn off the furnace.

THE ADRENAL-GLAND HORMONES

It is now time to get acquainted with the producers of cortisol in the human stress response, your adrenal glands. You have two of them, and they sit on top of each of your kidneys. The adrenal glands have two distinct parts: the innermost medulla, which comprises 20 percent of the gland, and the outer cortex. The adrenal medulla is related to the sympathetic nervous system, and its job is to secrete epinephrine and norepinephrine in response to sympathetic stimulation.

The cortex produces three types of hormones: mineralocorticoids, glucocorticoids (cortisol), and androgens. The mineralocorticoids affect the mineral content of the body and control the electrolytes, particularly sodium and potassium, in the body's extracellular fluids. The principal mineralocorticoid hormone is aldosterone.

The glucocorticoids (cortisol) get their name because of their effect on the concentration of glucose (sugar) in the blood. However, they also significantly affect both protein and fat metabolism. As we said, the principal glucocorticoid hormone is cortisol, and its ability to affect glucose, protein, and fat metabolism is all a part of its role in managing stress.

The androgenic hormones produced by the cortex play different roles, but they are largely considered to be sex hormones. The most important one is dehydroepiandrosterone, which fortunately for all of us has been abbreviated to DHEA. There have been a lot of things written about DHEA over the past several years, touting it as everything from the fountain of youth to the cure for cancer. The problem with most of these claims is that they fail to look at the bigger picture and how DHEA functions in a relative balance with cortisol. Taking oral doses of DHEA, which can be bought in any vitamin store, in the hope it will make you younger, sexier, or stronger without addressing an imbalance in cortisol levels is at best futile and at worst dangerous.

The reason DHEA received such notoriety as the "youth" hormone is because the adrenal glands produce the greatest quantities of it between the ages of seven and twenty-five. As we age, there is a progressive decline in DHEA production, and by age seventy-five, we are only producing 15 to 20 percent of what we were back in our peak years. So it is seductive to think that all you have to do is increase your levels of DHEA, and you will return to being the horny and crazy adolescent you once were. While this may be a great way to sell pills, it doesn't take into account the many factors that can cause DHEA production to be too low.

A very important feature of DHEA and cortisol secretion is that under normal circumstances they follow a predictable *circadian rhythm,* or twenty-four-hour cycle. Interestingly enough, this is also true of CRF (corticotrophin-releasing factor), secreted by the hypothalamus, and ACTH (adrenocorticotrophin hormone), secreted by the pituitary gland. The secretory levels of cortisol, CRF, and ACTH should be high in the early morning, peaking roughly around eight A.M. and then progressively declining until they reach their lowest level in the evening. The production of DHEA follows a daily, circadian cycle that is the opposite of cortisol, in order to maintain balance. As the cortisol levels should be declining throughout the day, the DHEA levels should be rising. This is important, because if your adrenal glands are producing elevated amounts of cortisol late at night, you will develop insomnia. You either will have trouble falling asleep, or, more typically, you will fall asleep just fine but find yourself waking up two and a half to three hours later and then have difficultly getting back to sleep. Sometimes you will lie awake staring at the ceiling for a half hour, and other times it will take several hours before you finally return to sleep.

This disruptive sleep pattern creates a twofold problem. The first one is the physiological and psychological consequence of sleep deprivation, which is fatigue and depression. The second problem is that your body conducts most of its repair functions while you are sleeping, and the inability to consistently restore worn or damaged cells will result in pain and illness.

The Human Stress Response

Let's follow an example of a stress response in the life of a typical human being living in a precivilized environment like New Jersey. You are walking around, minding your own business, looking for a few grubs or berries to eat, and you hear a sound like the snapping of a branch or the rustling of leaves.

Your body's first response is to have your thalamus evaluate the information it has just received. Maybe it's just the wind, or maybe it's a predator that thinks you might make a good lunch—and we are not talking about your culinary skills here. Your thalamus transfers this sensory information to your neocortex and the rest of your limbic system to "discuss" the significance of this stimulus. If they decide that danger is present, then you are hormonally off to the races, and I mean that literally. The next player on the team is the hypothalamus, which secretes the CRF that causes the pituitary gland to secrete ACTH, which in turn causes the cortex of the adrenal glands to secrete cortisol. Cortisol is such an elegantly effective global hormone that it can affect virtually every system in the body—an excellent way of orchestrating the body's expenditure of energy when survival is threatened. But as we will discover, the very thing that makes cortisol so concise and wonderful also makes it devastatingly dangerous when its levels are either too high or too low for prolonged periods of time.

Now back to lunch, where you are about to be the main course. You have now entered the moments of fight or flight, and either you are going to have a physical confrontation or you are going to try to outrun the predator and be a genetic ancestor of a future Boston marathon winner. The first thing you are going to need to accomplish either of these tasks is fuel, which in this case means sugar (glucose).

The release of cortisol will immediately stimulate a process known as *glucogenesis*. This is the formation of glucose from protein amino acids in the liver, and in a stress response, cortisol can increase the rate of glucose production by six to ten times the normal rate. This dramatically increases the availability of the fuel your muscles are going to need to get out of this dangerous predicament. However, to facilitate efficiency, your body has a unique mechanism for allowing the glucose to enter only those cells involved in the fight-or-flight response. The mechanism by which cortisol inhibits glucose from entering or being stored in certain cells during a stress response relies on the fact that cortisol counteracts the effects of insulin. As an additional part of the process, insulin production decreases when the sympathetic nervous system is activated.

Now we have the fuel delivery system, but we still need oxygen to make it work. It's time for cortisol to affect your cardiovascular system by narrowing your arteries while at the same time the epinephrine increases your heart rate. By pumping blood harder and faster through a narrower channel, you have increased your blood pressure and increased the flow of oxygen-enriched blood to your muscles. You have now mobilized the glucose and oxygen you need for the impending 100-yard dash or a few rounds with Mike Tyson's ancestor.

Why Elevated Levels of Cortisol Can Be Dangerous

While the secretion of cortisol orchestrates the response to stress and flips all of the right switches for fight or flight, the effects of cortisol

aren't quite done with you yet. In its infinite wisdom, your body figures that since, at this stressfully critical moment in time, your only
agenda is survival, it decides to shut down other functions that might
divert energy away from your fight-or-flight response or that simply
are not of value at this moment. One of the principal effects of cortisol on the metabolic systems of the body is the reduction of protein
stores in essentially all body cells except those of the liver. During the
stress response the protein amino acids in the liver are being converted to glucose for fuel, but everywhere else in the body either the
protein is being broken down through a process called *catabolism,* or
the synthesis of protein has stopped. Your body figures there is no
point in storing or making new protein if you are going to be dead in
two minutes, so it takes a wait-and-see approach. This means that
during a stress response your body will not engage in the growth or
repair processes of your tissues. As you can imagine, this can have dramatic repercussions if it goes on too long with chronic stress.

Cortisol and Sex

Another effect of elevated cortisol is the depletion of the reproductive system. Let's say you are a twenty-eight-year-old male being
chased by a predator, and you happen to run by a stream where young
women are bathing. Clearly, this is not the appropriate time to achieve
an erection. Your body is far more concerned about whether you will
still be alive in the next five minutes than whether you might be en-
gaging in sexual activity anytime in the near future, so it wisely sees
no point in facilitating the hormones of reproduction. If the stress goes
on for too long, a common repercussion among males is impotence.

   As for females, increased stress can both inhibit the libido and put
the brakes on the ovulating process. This can happen in several ways.
First, Jay Kaplan of Bowman Grey Medical School has demonstrated
that stress can suppress the estrogen levels of female monkeys as effectively as removing their ovaries. It also appears that while the adrenal
glands are busy producing cortisol and epinephrine for stress, they are
diverted from making the androgenic sex hormones. It is known that

the sex drive can be diminished by surgically removing the adrenal glands, and it can be restored with the administration of synthetic androgens.

Another facet of this complicated process for females is the adrenal androgen called androstenedione, the hormone that became famous when baseball player Mark McGuire ingested daily amounts of it in 1999 and hit a record number of home runs. In women, androstenedione is converted to estrogen by an enzyme in fat cells. Cortisol causes oxidation (burning) of fat cells for the purpose of converting the fatty acids into energy; coupled with chronic stress, this can cause the enzyme for estrogen to become depleted, resulting in hormonal imbalances. This is well documented with elite female athletes who simple stop having menstrual cycles because the intense physiological strain disrupts their normal hormonal balance.

Cortisol and the Immune System

Following the same apparent "logic" that applies to disarming your body's repair and reproductive systems during stress, the immune system is also inhibited as a part of the stress response. This occurs in several different ways, but mostly it is cortisol that is responsible for suppressing the immune system's ability to function.

On a very basic level, the immune system is comprised of white blood cells, called *lymphocytes* and *monocytes,* which are responsible for roaming around the body looking for infectious invading cells and foreign objects to attack and kill. There are also chemical messengers, called *interleukins,* which enable the white blood cells to communicate with each other and orchestrate the proper immune response.

How stress and, in particular, cortisol inhibit the immune system is a multifaceted issue. Cortisol can halt the maturation of white blood cells in the thymus gland and can even cause the thymus gland to shrink. Cortisol also suppresses the release of the interleukin messengers, which makes the white blood cells less responsive. And last, but certainly not least, cortisol can just flat out kill the white blood cells by entering them and destroying their DNA. Considering all of the ways stress can dismember the immune system, it's not hard to understand why people get sick after a period of stress. Nearly everyone can relate to the experience of getting sick after taking final exams or on their honeymoon or on vacation from a stressful job. There are many medical specialists who hold the view that cancer is prevalent twelve to eighteen months after a serious stress event has occurred.

Cortisol: The Body's Anti-inflammatory Agent

By now you probably think cortisol is the demon hormone that made that little girl's head spin around in *The Exorcist*, but it's not that simple. One of the positive effects of cortisol, other than potentially saving your behind in a fight-or-flight situation, is that it is a powerful anti-inflammatory agent. Understanding the relationship of cortisol to inflammation is critically important, and it is a big piece of the puzzle when things really go awry in the body.

When tissues are damaged or degraded by trauma, infections, or substances such as the prolonged use of nonsteriodal anti-inflammatory medications, antibiotic drugs, alcohol, caffeine, phosphoric acid (some sodas), or a diet that is high in omega-6 oils (processed foods, fast foods, and junk foods, which cause elevated levels of inflammatory prostaglandins), they almost always become inflamed. In some cases, such as rheumatoid arthritis, the inflammation is the most damaging part of the disease. When tissues become inflamed, a damaging cascade of events occurs. The damaged tissue cells release chemicals, such as histamine, proteolytic enzymes, and prostaglandins, that initiate the inflammatory response.

As an example that is easy to relate to, let's take your nose. Your darling child comes home from preschool as a carrier of every germ known to the National Institutes of Health and gives you a big hug and a kiss. These germs now enter your system either orally or as airborne messengers of disease. If your immune system is not up to the challenge, these microbes will set up camp in your throat or nasal passage and begin to multiply. At some point, specialized cells of your immune system, called *mast cells,* will become aware of the invading organisms, yell "Mayday! Mayday!" and then explode. The purpose of this is to release histamine, which will cause inflammation in order to attract the white blood cells of your immune system, and so launch the holy war in your mucous membranes. This is when, with tissues in hand, you head for the drugstore in search of antihistamine nasal sprays or pills to reduce the inflammation and swelling.

As we have already discussed, cortisol can suppress the immune system. At first you might think this is a stupid act on your body's part and no wonder your cold seems to last for weeks. Here you are taking echinacea, goldenseal, and God knows what else to build up your immune system, and those knuckleheaded adrenal glands are producing cortisol to suppress it. Well, this is where the importance of homeostasis or balance comes in.

Cortisol affects inflammation in several ways. Cortisol stabilizes the membranes of the cells that release the proteolytic enzymes, histamines, and prostaglandins that cause inflammation. Furthermore, by reducing the permeability of the small blood vessels, cortisol restricts the transport of these inflammatory chemicals throughout the body. An example of cortisol's powerful effect on inflammation, especially if you have ever had poison ivy or poison oak rashes, is the prescription drug called *cortisone,* which is pharmaceutically manufactured cortisol.

An unchecked immune system responding to unabated inflammation will probably eat you up over time and turn into an autoimmune disease, as a result of which your immune system begins attacking normal cells. So in appropriate amounts, cortisol acts as damage control by reducing the inflammation and also by not allowing the immune system to get overly aggressive. In a similar vein (no pun intended), the reduction in permeability of the small blood vessels reduces the migration of the white blood cells throughout the body, which again regulates the immune response.

Another aspect of cortisol's participation in the immune response is that it can lower fever by inhibiting the release of interleukin-1, which besides being an immune messenger is also the chemical that excites the hypothalamic temperature control. Having a fever when you are sick is a great defense mechanism, because it is your body's way of trying to create an environment that the invading microbes can't live in. But in the wisdom of homeostasis and in an effort to not cook your brain cells, cortisol can keep this process from getting out of control.

There is no doubt that proper levels of cortisol are crucial to or-chestrating the appropriate response to life-threatening stress or to managing inflammation and the immune system. But what happens if the stress (physical, psychological, or a combination of both) becomes chronic, or the inflammation becomes chronic, or the stress and the inflammation get caught up in a vicious dance with each other?

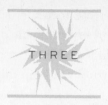

THREE

PHYSICAL STRESS AND
THE PRO-INFLAMMATORY DIET

There's a Fire Down Below

I n its classic interpretation, physical stress is usually correlated with the fight-or-flight survival response. However, other physical stressors, such as pain and, more important, inflammation, cause cortisol levels to become elevated to the point at which they can become chronic and dangerous. Inflammation and the damage it causes to the body have been ignored for far too long by the medical community, but recent research has shown how serious inflammation can be, and new federal recommendations are being written that urge doctors to test for it. In fact, inflammation is now attracting a great deal of attention from medical researchers who consider it to be an even bigger factor in heart disease than cholesterol. In a research paper published in the *New England Journal of Medicine* on November 14, 2002, Dr. Paul Ridker of Boston's Brigham and Women's Hospital states that up to 35 million Americans have normal cholesterol but above-average levels of inflammation, putting them at unusual risk for heart attacks and strokes.

CAUSES OF INFLAMMATION

Interestingly enough, this article never determines where all of this inflammation is coming from, but it is my contention that chronic intestinal-tract inflammation caused by the overuse of nonsteroidal anti-inflammatory drugs (NSAIDs), caffeinated beverages, alcohol, antibiotics, mental stress, or any combination of these factors is a significant piece of this puzzle. The other cause of inflammation is going to be the pro-inflammatory diet, in which the consumption of foods high in omega-6 oils causes elevated levels of prostaglandin-E2, which is a highly inflammatory chemical. Sadly, this describes the typical American diet of fast foods, junk foods, fried foods, and processed foods. While intestinal-tract inflammation is *specific* to one organ, the pro-inflammatory diet results in *systemic* inflammation, meaning that there is a highly inflammatory chemical circulating through the bloodstream. I think the medical researchers involved with inflammation are in a quandary regarding the revelation of the causes of inflammation, as they are probably not thrilled about taking on either the pharmaceutical or fast-food industries.

Remember, the human response to stress is designed to handle short-term stress, since all of the biochemical processes are clearly meant for managing a fight-or-flight response. After all, just how long do you think it takes to either run from or fight a tiger? It obviously does not benefit the survival of a species to develop a mechanism for stress management that can shut down its own repair and growth processes, reproductive functions, and immune system if it wasn't designed with the intention that the stress would be relatively short-term.

The Beginning of Trouble

So how does the physical stress of inflammation or injury cause elevated levels of stress hormones? I want to take you now through a few scenarios that occur with alarming regularity and illustrate how cortisol imbalances get started, how they can spiral out of control, and how devastating is their effect on human health.

You lift something improperly, spend too much time in the garden bent over pulling weeds, slip and fall down, get into a car accident, or injure yourself in a sporting activity, and now you are in pain. The pain isn't going away as quickly as you had hoped, and as a good, television-abiding American you want "fast, fast, fast relief." You go to your medicine cabinet and choose from any number of nonsteroidal anti-inflammatory drugs (NSAIDs) that are lined up on the shelves. There are an amazing number of NSAIDs available, of which the most popular are:

Ibuprofen (e.g., Motrin, Advil)
Aspirin (e.g., Bayer, Anacin, Bufferin)
Naproxen (e.g., Aleve, Anaprox)
Piroxicam (e.g., Feldene)
Sulindac (e.g., Clinoril)
Diclofenac (e.g., Voltaren)

An exception to this list is acetaminophen (Tylenol), which is an analgesic pain reliever that does not affect inflammation.

NSAIDs relieve inflammation in much the same way cortisol does: by blocking the release of prostaglandins and arachidonic acid. So far, so good. But what if your injury does not improve, and you continue to take them for an extended period of time?

There are several research studies that have looked into this question, and their conclusions are staggering. Swiss researchers report that NSAIDs are killing at least 2,000 patients each year in the United Kingdom because of bleeding ulcers. The researchers say that NSAIDs block the production of a coenzyme (cox-1) that protects the mucous lining of the stomach. This study suggests that about 1 in 1,000 patients who take these drugs regularly for two years will die from them.

A study published by Stanford University School of Medicine in April 1999 paints an even darker picture. This study states: "Nonsteroidal anti-inflammatory drugs are one of the most commonly used classes of medications worldwide. It is estimated that more than 30 million people take NSAIDs daily. Gastrointestinal inflammation related to NSAID therapy is the most prevalent category of adverse drug reactions." The statistics that this Stanford study reveals are truly alarming:

- In this country, 103,000 people are hospitalized yearly due to intestinal-tract inflammation caused by NSAIDs, at an average cost of $15,000 to $20,000 per case.
- An average of 16,500 deaths occur in the United States every year from intestinal-tract inflammation and bleeding caused by NSAIDs compared to this country's yearly rate of 16,685 deaths caused by HIV (human immunodeficiency virus).
- If NSAID-related deaths were tabulated separately in the National Vital Statistics report, it would be the fifteenth most common cause of death in the United States, putting it far ahead of deaths caused by Hodgkin's disease, ovarian cancer, and asthma.
- Only one out of five people who have serious intestinal-tract inflammation will have any warning signs.

Now here comes the really scary part: The statistics from this Stanford study account only for people who have been prescribed NSAIDs by their medical doctors for arthritis. The study did not take into account all of the people who regularly take over-the-counter NSAIDs for headaches, back pain, or other pain syndromes.

By examining the effects of NSAIDs on the digestive tract we can see the origin of the adrenal dilemma. You are in pain, which means there is likely to be some degree of inflammation involved, and you are taking NSAIDs. However, because the NSAIDs are only treating the symptoms and not the cause of your pain, the pain persists, and you continue to take the NSAIDs to relieve your symptoms. The NSAIDs are now inhibiting the prostaglandin production you need to repair your digestive tract on a daily basis from the onslaught of acids and enzymes necessary to digest your food. As the protective mucous lining of your digestive tract becomes degraded, the walls of the tract become inflamed, so now you have even more inflammation in your body than you started with.

Can you just guess what your adrenal glands are up to by now? You will recall that the adrenal glands will produce cortisol in any stress response, including tissue injury and inflammation. Cortisol, like NSAIDs, also inhibits the production of the prostaglandins that repair the digestive tract, so at this point the inflammation in your digestive tract is going to get progressively worse, causing even higher levels of cortisol to be produced, which will simply exacerbate the problem. You have begun the odyssey into the nightmare of chronic adrenal stress, a vicious cycle of pain, increased cortisol levels, the inability to repair tissue damage and inflammation, and more pain.

Leaky-Gut Syndrome

After your gastrointestinal tract has been inflamed for several months and the tissue lining has become progressively eroded, the next step in this process is the occurrence of microscopic holes in the intestinal wall, which will cause the wall to become abnormally porous and to leak incompletely digested bits of food, microbes, and toxins into your system. Commonly referred to as *leaky-gut syndrome,* a condition in which metabolic and microbial toxins escape from the small intestines and flood into the bloodstream, it has at least two negative consequences.

The first consequence of leaky-gut syndrome is that the incompletely digested particles of food and microbes escaping from the small intestinal lining will trigger an immune-system response. Any time a foreign object enters the body, it is the responsibility of the immune system to attack it, and most of the time this process works efficiently. With leaky-gut syndrome, the immune system perceives these escaping food particles as dangerous viruses and mounts an attack. At the same time, viruses and bacteria are also leaking out of the intestines, and the immune system is going to have to deal with them as well. This puts a continuous strain on the immune system, and the immune-system response becomes an exercise in futility because, as long as the intestinal tract is leaking and you keep eating, your immune system is never going to be able to get ahead of the toxins.

To help complicate matters further, the adrenal glands are still producing elevated levels of cortisol in response to the intestinal-tract inflammation and, as we discussed in the previous chapter, cortisol works to suppress the immune system. If this goes on for a prolonged period of time, the immune system will begin to break down.

The second negative consequence of leaky-gut syndrome concerns the liver's ability to detoxify your body. Think of your liver as a waste-management treatment plant that is responsible for screening out all of the junk circulating in your body. This process is called *stage two detoxification,* and it works as follows: All of the blood circulating in the body must pass through the liver before it returns to the lungs and heart. As the blood passes through, the liver removes toxic waste material. If the toxins are water soluble, the kidneys are responsible for excreting them in the urine. If they are fat soluble, the liver shunts the toxins through the common bile duct of the gallbladder, which is located directly under the liver, and the bile duct carries the toxins to the small intestinal tract. The toxins that end up in the intestinal tract will then be processed by a combination of digestive enzymes and healthy microbes and then eliminated in a bowel movement.

But remember, in this scenario the wall of the intestinal tract has microscopic holes in it and cannot contain the toxins being transported to it by the liver, resulting in a toxic merry-go-round. The very toxins that the liver is trying to remove keep circulating back to it over and over again, thereby creating continuous stress on the liver and gallbladder duct.

At this stage you are experiencing some sort of pain that has become chronic, be it headaches, neck or lower back pain, or some other joint pain. As you will recall from Chapter 2, the normal secretion of cortisol follows a daily circadian rhythm in which the cortisol level is highest in the morning and lowest at night. Elevated levels of cortisol at night result in insomnia. So now your body can't repair itself very well because the elevated levels of cortisol are suppressing your body's natural repair mechanisms *and* disrupting your normal sleep, which is the time your body should be carrying out the repair process.

So, your digestive tract is inflamed from all of the NSAIDs you are taking and leaking all manner of toxins into your bloodstream, and your immune system is being suppressed and overworked at the same time. You aren't sleeping at night, and you are probably craving sugar, salt, or both, due to cortisol's effect on inhibiting your insulin and weakening the adrenal sodium/potassium pump, which regulates your body's mineral content. Your life is not exactly wonderful.

You have plenty of physical problems, which by now are probably causing some mental stress. You don't feel well, and you are beginning to worry that maybe you are never going to feel well ever again. You are not sleeping well because the elevation of cortisol causes you to wake up around two o'clock in the morning, and you toss and turn for an hour or more before you can get back to sleep, so now you are tired and cranky to boot. Your blood sugar is bouncing up and down, which makes you crave and eat foods that end up making you feel even worse. You are gaining weight as a result of eating the carbohydrates you are craving and because you can't exercise due to the pain you are experiencing. You are also experiencing mood swings, and you are either easily agitated and argumentative, or withdrawn and depressed, or both at varying times.

Given the fact that you are run down and your immune system is overtaxed, the next misfortune you are likely to encounter is that you begin getting sick more often with colds, influenza, or other infections. This will bring you to your medical doctor and a probable course of antibiotic therapy.

The problem with antibiotics is that they destroy the beneficial bacteria living in your small and large intestines. The intestinal tract has over five hundred different kinds of beneficial bacteria that perform hundreds of functions for a healthy metabolism and immune response. Through enzyme secretions, bacteria transform metabolic and microbial wastes before they are discharged in a bowel movement. If you already have an inflamed intestinal tract from too many NSAIDs, and subsequent leaky-gut syndrome, taking antibiotics will only further impair your ability to purge toxins from your system.

If all of this is happening to you and you happen to be a woman, you are likely to experience even further complications in your hormonal balance because the amount of estrogen that gets released into your system is regulated by the liver and the bacteria in the intestinal tract. The liver sends excess estrogen through the gallbladder duct to the small intestines, where the normal bacteria break it down. If you lack the bacteria to destroy excess estrogen and you have intestinal leakage, the estrogen will be reabsorbed and can end up in estrogen-receptor sites such as the breasts, ovaries, and uterus. This may contribute to fibroid tumors, estrogen-sensitive cancers, premenstrual syndrome (PMS), and monthly migraines related to menstrual cycles.

Candida Yeast Infections

Should you continue on either a prolonged or repetitive course of antibiotic therapy, you will graduate to another problem, which is a Candida infection in the intestinal tract. *Candida albicans* is a yeast that, under normal circumstances, inhabits the intestinal tract in relative balance with the rest of the intestinal microbes. Unfortunately, the antibiotics will kill the normal bacteria that serve to keep the Candida population in check. The Candida cells excrete a chemical that shrinks the cells of the intestinal wall, and as these cells continue to wither away, the intestinal tract further degrades, becomes more inflamed, and leaks even more toxins into the bloodstream.

So now you have a Candida infection, and the yeast is living off the carbohydrates you are eating, which results in a further imbalance in your blood-sugar levels. Remember that an elevated level of cortisol will inhibit your cells' sensitivity to insulin and your ability to store glucose for energy; now the Candida is living off your glucose-producing foods before you can even use them, and your energy level is dropping because your muscles and brain are starved for the glucose that fuels them. Your sugar cravings are increasing; you are consuming lots of junk food that is high in calories; and you are probably gaining more weight.

You obviously are still not getting well. You still have pain; you seem to get sick every other week; and your friends, loved ones, and the people you work with are starting to think you are a hypochondriac. You are missing work because of your multiple illnesses, and when you are there, you are not very productive. But at least things can't get any worse. Or can they?

Autoimmune Attacks

This is a good time to recall that cortisol suppresses the part of the immune system that is responsible for preventing an autoimmune attack. How your immune system knows which cells belong to you and which ones don't, and therefore are worthy of killing, is called "self-tolerance," a process regulated by cells produced in the thymus gland and bone marrow. Prolonged periods of elevated cortisol levels can destroy immune-system cells, rob these cells of the chemicals that are necessary for them to function properly, and even *shrink* the thymus gland that is making these immune-system cells. Add this to the fact that your poor immune system is already overburdened by dealing with the toxins leaking out of your intestinal tract, and this might provide an excellent opportunity to develop an autoimmune disease. The overworked, poorly formed immune cells begin to make mistakes and start attacking the body's own tissues, resulting in diseases such as rheumatoid arthritis, fibromyalgia, thyroid disease, and multiple sclerosis. I will discuss autoimmune diseases in greater detail a little later when we delve into cortisol's role in specific diseases.

Adrenal Fatigue

This brings us to the other side of the problem with adrenal-gland disorders, which is that it is not always a matter of producing too *much* cortisol but too *little*. This is known as *adrenal fatigue,* and it is the last phase of adrenal maladaptation. In the first phase the cortisol levels are too high, and the DHEA levels are normal; in the second phase the cortisol levels are still too high, but the DHEA levels are now too low; and in the final phase the adrenal glands are worn out and incapable of making appropriate amounts of hormones, causing both the cortisol and DHEA levels to be too low.

A deficiency in cortisol will make it impossible to maintain normal blood-sugar levels throughout the day. Cortisol is necessary for a process known as *glucogenesis,* which is the conversion of proteins into usable glucose (sugar), and an abnormal reduction of cortisol results in lowered blood-sugar levels. This is a clear example of why it is so important for the cortisol levels to be normal, because if they are too high, cortisol inhibits insulin utilization so that you can't metabolize the carbohydrates you eat into usable glucose, and if they are too low, you can't convert proteins into glucose. Either way your blood sugar is too low, which all by itself can cause fatigue, headaches, irritability, and sugar cravings.

Another effect of insufficient cortisol is the inability to access proteins and fats from the body's tissues, which depresses many other metabolic functions. This creates a sluggish metabolism even if plenty of glucose and nutrients are otherwise available to the muscles. The lack of cortisol will make the muscles weak and dysfunctional.

Inadequate cortisol secretion also makes the body more susceptible to the deteriorating effects of stress, increasing the likelihood of infections and difficulty in getting over them. Once again, this is an excellent example of the need for homeostasis or balance; too much or too little cortisol has a negative effect on the immune system. This is one of those chicken or egg situations: Are you stressed out because you are sick, or are you sick because you are stressed?

While people with cortisol levels that are too high have a hair-trigger response to stress and fly off the handle with the least bit of provocation, people whose cortisol levels are too low are also unable to deal with stress appropriately and are easily overwhelmed. They are *literally* sick and tired, and the simple tasks of everyday life become magnified into problems they can't deal with. Their sodium and glucose levels are unstable, causing them to crave salt and/or sugar; their muscles are getting progressively weaker; their immune system is going further downhill; and their ability to have a normal and productive life is seriously compromised. This is the point where chronic fatigue syndrome is likely to occur.

DIET, INFLAMMATION, AND HORMONE IMBALANCE

The inability to recover from an injury or to resolve a pain syndrome, the repetitive use of NSAIDs, and the overuse of antibiotics are not the only ways to end up with imbalanced cortisol levels. Another scenario is that of a chronically poor diet, which can adversely disturb hormonal function by directly affecting the ability of the adrenal glands to function normally or cause systemic inflammation by elevating the levels of arachidonic acid and trigger its conversion to prostaglandin-E2 (PG-E2). PG-E2 is such a potent inflammatory chemical that it is considered to be the biological equivalent of putting gasoline on a fire.

Poor diet can be a major player in causing hormonal imbalances, and it can do so on several levels. Pumping your body full of caffeine with coffee, tea, soda, or chocolate will jolt your adrenal glands and mimic a stress response. The acidity of caffeinated beverages can also disturb the lining of the intestinal tract and result in inflammation. Consuming large amounts of alcohol will damage the intestinal tract, upset your blood-sugar levels, stress your liver, and ultimately act as a stimulant.

Eating more than a moderate amount of sugar will obviously distort your blood sugar, and since cortisol is the body's antidote to elevated insulin, it is likely that your cortisol levels will rise. If you eat a lot of sugar and fast foods, you are depriving the adrenal glands of the nutrients they need from fresh fruits and vegetables to function properly. (The adrenal glands require more vitamin C than any other tissue of the body.) You also stand a good chance of gaining weight, and as your weight increases, you are less likely to exercise. Exercise is very helpful in keeping your adrenal glands balanced, and it is a good way to get the stress of everyday life out of your system.

Another negative consequence of eating too much sugar or processed foods that convert easily to sugar is that it causes the pancreas to keep pumping out insulin, to the point where the oversecretion of insulin results in low blood sugar (hypoglycemia). As the pancreas is trying desperately to keep the level of blood sugar normal in the face of a constant barrage of sugar consumption, it can oversecrete insulin and pull too much sugar out of the bloodstream. The end result is low blood sugar and the further craving for sugar, which perpetuates the cycle over and over again.

A pro-inflammatory diet is one that is so high in hydrogenated oils, trans-fatty acids, and saturated fats that it will increase levels of prostaglandin-E2 (PG-E2) to the point where systemic inflammation occurs. These oils and fats occur in nearly every form of fast food; processed foods such as crackers, cookies, donuts, and baked goods; and anything made with corn oil. These oils are in the omega-6 class of fats, and they cause the conversion of arachidonic acid to PG-E2, which then circulates throughout the body as an inflammatory chemical. Since we all know by now what the body's response to inflammation is, we can expect an elevation of cortisol with all of the potential problems that come with it.

There is one last, very serious problem with a diet high in omega-6 fats regarding hormonal balance, and that is its effect on the actual receptor sites on every cell in the body. Neurotransmitters, such as serotonin and dopamine, polypeptides, hormones, and amino acids (which means virtually every chemical a cell needs to function normally), need to be able to attach to specific receptor sites in order to effect cellular function. The receptors are made of protein and are embedded in a lipid (fat) membrane that makes up the outer wall of each cell. If the lipid wall is soft (in neuroscience the terms used are *fluid* or *plastic*), then the neurotransmitters can easily dock on to the receptors. However, if the lipid wall becomes hard and less fluid, the shape of the receptor site changes, and the neurotransmitters cannot adequately attach to the receptors, or in other words, the cell becomes physiologically impaired. The consequences of this situation on human health are enormous and can result in depression (serotonin inhibition), Parkinson's disease (dopamine inhibition), and any number of hormonal imbalances because the hormones simply cannot communicate with the cells, leading to a host of symptoms.

The scenarios I have been describing here are not uncommon, and doctors' offices are filled with patients whose health problems are spiraling out of control. As doctors are trained to treat specific symptoms with specific drugs, these patients can quickly find themselves on a myriad of medications for insomnia, depression, pain, and gastric upset that fail to address the *causal* factors of their health problems, namely intestinal-tract inflammation, a pro-inflammatory diet, and cortisol imbalances. In the upcoming chapters, I will show you how to accurately test your cortisol levels, resolve intestinal-tract and systemic inflammation, restore hormonal balance, and get you on the road to regaining your health.

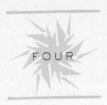

FOUR

TESTING
CORTISOL LEVELS

The Conditions for Murder Are Met

f your health status resembles what I have been describing in the preceding chapters, then it is very probable that your cortisol levels are out of balance. If you are having trouble sleeping, find yourself craving sugar and/or salt, and you are irritable and feel overwhelmed most of the time, then your cortisol levels are unstable. But it is not enough to assume that your cortisol levels are out of balance; we need to know *when* they are out of balance and by *how much*.

Fortunately, there is an easy and highly accurate way to find out just what your adrenal glands are doing throughout the day using a method known as *salivary testing*. Steroid hormones enter the saliva through passive diffusion of the soft tissue of the saliva glands. From there the hormones can be tested by taking saliva samples at precise times of the day to see how well the adrenal glands are adapting to stress.

The National Aeronautics and Space Administration (NASA) is now using salivary testing to measure the cortisol levels of its astronauts. One of the serious obstacles to lengthy space missions is the stress of confinement in a small capsule with seven other people for nine months, as would be the case during a trip to Mars. Astronauts who have spent several months aboard the space station *Mir* have warned NASA that the claustrophobic conditions could easily result in a homicide. So in an effort to avoid what would be a very embarrassing "Houston, we have a problem" communiqué, NASA has employed cortisol testing.

The Adrenal Stress Index

The salivary test for adrenal function is called the adrenal stress index (ASI), and it is done in the comfort of your home or workplace over the period of one day. It is a test kit that has four vials for the collection of saliva samples. Each vial is labeled for the time the sample should be collected, which is morning, noon, late afternoon (five P.M. to six P.M.), and midnight.

After collecting a sample in the appropriate vial, it is stored in the refrigerator, and after all of the samples have been taken, you ship them to the laboratory via overnight mail. There are several laboratories that can evaluate these tests (see the Resource Guide at the end of book), and two of the best are the Great Smokies Laboratory and Diagnos-Techs., Inc. The test results are sent back to your doctor with detailed graphs that chart your cortisol/DHEA levels and ratios.

The adrenal stress index test also measures something called *gliadin antibodies SigA,* which detects an allergic reaction in the intestinal wall to wheat, rye, oat, and other grains that contain gluten. This can be very useful as a marker for intestinal-tract inflammation and Candida infections.

In the previous chapters we went through the symptomatic downward spiraling of adrenal-gland maladaptation to stress, be it psychological, physiological, or both. There are technically four phases of response to stress that the adrenal glands can exhibit, and they are:

Phase 1. *The Normal Stress Response*

The limbic system, which is the part of your brain that manages stress, perceives a physical or emotional stressor and, as you will remember, initiates a chain of hormone secretions. The hypothalamus secretes CRF, which causes the pituitary to secrete ACTH, and this signals the adrenal glands to release cortisol and DHEA. As the stressful situation unfolds, the cortisol and DHEA will rise in a balanced ratio and set in motion all of the physiological changes necessary in an attempt to successfully deal with the stress. If the stress is resolved, the cortisol signals the limbic system to stop secreting the ACTH, which, in turn, stops the cortisol production. As the cortisol levels return to normal, the physiological changes your body went through during the stress also return to normal.

Phase 2. *The Compensated/Divergence Phase*

When the stress or inflammation has become chronic and the cortisol levels have been elevated for an extended period of time, you've reached the second phase. Keep in mind that stress affects individuals differently, and the time frame that constitutes "chronic stress" for one person can be quite different for another. Another factor to be considered is the intensity of the stress. If you just found out that your wife has cancer and you've just lost your job, the stress is going to be far more profound, and you may get to this compensated/divergence phase far sooner than someone whose cortisol levels are rising as a result of progressive intestinal-tract inflammation.

Compensated refers to what happens in the hypothalamus and pituitary glands when the cortisol levels remain elevated, and these glands compensate by becoming less sensitive to the cortisol. The reason for this, as we will see more clearly when we get to the next phase, is that cortisol can damage these brain cells, and the hypothalamus and pituitary glands compensate and try to protect their cells by becoming less sensitive to cortisol. However, this decrease in sensitivity weakens the negative feedback loop that tells the hypothalamus to stop secreting CRF and, therefore, halt the pituitary gland's secretion of ACTH. Since it is the ACTH that signals the adrenal glands to produce cortisol, the pituitary gland's inability to stop secreting ACTH means that cortisol production can't be turned off. It is here where the beginning of insomnia may kick in, especially where falling asleep is not so difficult, but you wake up in the middle of the night because of the failure of the pituitary gland to keep the cortisol levels within its normal circadian rhythms.

Divergence refers to what happens when the cortisol levels are still high, but the adrenal glands are no longer able to keep up the production of DHEA as they did in the normal stress response, so that the cortisol and DHEA levels begin to pull away in different directions. The adrenal glands are still producing DHEA, but not at the same rate they were able to before the stress became more chronic.

It is in this compensated/divergence phase that your cells' sensitivity to insulin and glucose is impaired, since cortisol inhibits glucose storage, and your blood-sugar levels are bouncing around. Cravings for sugar are likely to occur, and fat accumulation around the waist may be increasing. Along with a decline in DHEA production, the adrenal glands may not be adequately producing other hormones, like the mineralocorticoids that maintain mineral balance. This will cause you to crave salt and/or magnesium because these minerals are being overly excreted in your urine. The most common response to a lowering of magnesium in the bloodstream is to crave chocolate, which is very high in magnesium. In the case of cravings for salt, most people unfortunately gravitate toward things like potato or corn chips, which are high in both poor-quality carbohydrates that promote sugar cravings and fats that cause systemic inflammation.

Phase 3. The Decompensated/Maladaptive Phase

At this point, your cortisol levels are still elevated, but now there is an abnormal decline in DHEA production. The hypothalamus and pituitary glands that were previously compensating for the elevated levels of cortisol are now becoming less and less able to protect themselves from the ravaging effects of being continuously bombarded by cortisol. In laboratory experiments, cortisol has been proven to damage and kill brain cells in the limbic system. The ability of the hypothalamus, pituitary, and adrenal glands to adapt and communicate with each other is declining (hence the term *maladaptive*), and so is your health.

Your symptoms are now becoming more intense, and everything is getting worse: the insomnia, lowered energy levels, more intense food cravings, a weakened immune system, mood swings and/or depression.

Phase 4. The Fatigue Phase

Now the bottom has fallen out, and there is minimal feedback sensitivity to cortisol in the limbic system, but it doesn't matter because the adrenal glands are burned out and unable to produce much cortisol at all. The DHEA levels are actually higher than the cortisol levels, but they are still abnormally low, and you are excessively fatigued, depressed, have an inability to concentrate and think clearly, and have a great potential for degenerative diseases.

It is precisely because the adrenal glands have these different phases, and because these phases and symptoms can overlap a bit depending on individual lifestyles (a person with a good diet and exercise regime is likely to hold up better than someone without them), that salivary testing is so important. Clearly, unless your doctor knows exactly where your level of adrenal-gland malfunction is, you will not get the proper treatment.

BLOOD TESTS VERSUS SALIVA TESTS

Many doctors do not yet understand the importance of measuring cortisol levels, and those who do often rely on a blood test. Unfortunately, there are three problems in trying to assess cortisol levels in this manner. The first problem is that a person's cortisol level may be fine during one part of the day but imbalanced during another part of the day. For example, it is not unusual for me to see an adrenal stress index test where the cortisol level is fine in the morning, too low in the afternoon, and then too high late at night. Any combination of these imbalances throughout the day can and do occur, so trying to accurately measure cortisol levels with a single blood sample taken at whatever time of the day you happen to see your doctor is not going to be very revealing as to the whole scope of your problem.

The second problem is that some people become nervous in a doctor's office, to such an extent that their blood pressure goes up and causes inaccurate readings when their blood pressure is taken. This is known as "white coat syndrome," and if it can elevate a person's blood pressure, then it will certainly elevate his or her cortisol levels and yield inaccurate results.

The third problem with using a blood test is that it will reflect the *total* hormone level and not what is called the *unbound bioactive fraction*, which is the actual hormone level on which the living cells are actually functioning. In this way, blood-serum testing is not very reflective of what is really happening inside of your body.

Since 1983, more than 2,500 scientific papers and research articles pertaining to salivary diagnostic testing have been published, yet salivary testing has still not come into mainstream medical practice. Many hormonal profiles can be tested in addition to adrenal gland function: e.g., female hormone levels, both pre- and postmenopausal; testosterone; thyroid hormones; glucose and insulin levels; and gluten (wheat) intolerance and immune-system function.

One of my goals in writing this book is to make salivary adrenal testing as routine as all the other diagnostic tests that patients take in their annual physical examinations. If your doctor is so concerned about your glucose and cholesterol levels, then why not be equally concerned about your cortisol levels? Should your doctor express no interest in checking your adrenal-gland function, the resources section at the end of the book will guide you to doctors who are familiar and competent in interpreting adrenal stress indexes and other salivary tests.

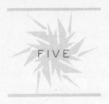

THE RELATIONSHIP OF CORTISOL
TO OTHER DISEASES

The Missing Link

In the beginning of this book I gave you a virtual laundry list of diseases and disorders that can be caused by cortisol imbalance. Perhaps the reason you have chosen to read this book is because you have one of these health problems and either are hoping to better understand its causal factors or would like to learn other approaches to managing it. As an easy reference guide, I am going to summarize each one of these disorders and explain the involvement of cortisol and DHEA imbalances.

HEART DISEASE

One of the facets of the human response to stress is the constriction of the blood vessels in order to increase the delivery of oxygenated blood; their continuous constriction due to chronic stress can result in damage and plaque buildup. This occurs because the constriction and increased blood pressure against the wall of the artery can cause the layers of the vessel to break down. Your arteries have three layers, and the innermost one is very smooth, so that all the round blood cells can roll through the arteries quickly. The middle layer of the artery is sticky in order to hold the inner and outer layers together. The compromise in this wonderful design occurs where a larger artery bifurcates, or divides, to become smaller arteries. It is at this juncture that the increase in blood pressure, continually pounding away at this dividing point, weakens the inner wall and causes it to peel away.

As the inner layer becomes degraded, the middle sticky layer becomes exposed. This allows the fats, starches, and calcium floating around in the bloodstream to adhere to the flypaperlike surface. Over a prolonged period of time this will result in the buildup of plaque found in heart disease and atherosclerosis (hardening of the arteries). As the plaque becomes thicker, it blocks the artery and restricts blood flow to the muscular wall of the heart. By choking off the flow of oxygenated blood, the cells of the heart muscle progressively die, and thus the stage is set for a heart attack (myocardial infarction).

We have been led to believe that heart disease is attributable to high-fat diets and elevated levels of cholesterol. However, this is not completely accurate, as shown by research done by physiologist Jay Kaplan of Bowman Gray Medical School. Kaplan has proven that social stress alone can cause atherosclerosis and high blood pressure in mice and primates and that this can occur even with a low-fat diet.

It is not only arterial plaques and restricted blood flow that can cause heart attacks, but also arterial spasms induced by strong emotional states, especially anger. Researchers at the University of North Carolina have published a study that finds a threefold increase in the frequency of heart attacks in people who are prone to fits of anger. This is related to the fact that cortisol constricts blood vessels.

Higher levels of cortisol have been found in people with heart disease, and lower concentrations of DHEA were recorded in young men who had heart attacks due to atherosclerosis. It is important to remember that cortisol imbalances precede DHEA imbalances because the DHEA levels don't begin to decline until the adrenal glands have reached the decompensated/maladaptive stage. DHEA was found to be significantly reduced in the urine of people with high blood pressure (hypertension) when compared to those with normal blood pressure.

DIABETES

Diabetes mellitus is the fourth leading cause of death in the United States and it comes in two varieties.

The first type is *insulin-dependent diabetes mellitus* (IDDM), which refers to the inability of the cells of the pancreas to produce adequate amounts of insulin on demand. This type comprises only between 5 and 10 percent of all diabetes cases and one risk factor is thought to be genetic. As the name implies, people with IDDM are dependent on insulin as a necessary part of their treatment. Depending on the severity of the diabetes, the insulin may be taken orally in pill form, or it may require injections to keep blood-sugar levels stable.

The second type of diabetes is called *non-insulin-dependent diabetes mellitus* (NIDDM), and it makes up the other 90 to 95 percent of diabetics. The number of people with this type of diabetes is staggering, and the incidence of it has risen almost 50 percent since 1983. Nearly 6 percent of Americans have this type of diabetes, and there is an average of 798,000 new cases each year. In this type of diabetes, the pancreas is actually making insulin, but the cells have become desensitized, or resistant to the insulin.

Insulin resistance means that the receptor sites on the cell walls that are supposed to have an affinity to insulin to allow glucose to enter the cells are now resistant to the insulin. Being resistant to your own insulin is about the same as not producing insulin: Either way, you cannot effectively utilize glucose. However, in this case, your pancreas responds to the resistance by producing more insulin, and while this doesn't help in glucose utilization, it does seriously raise the level of triglycerides in your system, thereby increasing the risk of heart disease. To make matters worse, insulin signals the liver to make more cholesterol, so as the pancreas keeps secreting more insulin in response to your resistance, your cholesterol levels keep rising.

One of the principal functions of cortisol is to counteract the effects of insulin, because in fight-or-flight stress you don't want to store energy; you need to mobilize energy immediately to meet life-threatening demands. One of the ways cortisol accomplishes this is by making your cells resistant to insulin, which for short-term stress management is appropriate. When the cortisol level remains chronically elevated, however, it can become a factor in non-insulin-dependent diabetes mellitus, as long-term insulin resistance sets in and the pancreas struggles to produce ever-escalating quantities of insulin.

Insomnia

In a properly functioning system, cortisol secretion follows a definite circadian rhythm, with highest levels typically occurring at eight o'clock in the morning and progressively declining throughout the day until reaching very low levels late at night. Since the function of cortisol is to create a state of alertness and arousal as a necessary response to stress, elevated levels of cortisol at night will obviously cause insomnia.

There are two types of insomnia, one in which you can't fall asleep to begin with, and the other, more common one, in which you have no problem falling asleep but are awake again after three or four hours and have trouble getting back to sleep.

Nearly everyone has experienced an episode of insomnia in his or her life because of an immediate stressor, such as worrying about an exam, a job interview, or some unpleasant situation that needs to be resolved. In the normal response to stress, these short-term episodes resolve as the stressful situation passes.

If the cause of the insomnia is psychological stress of a more serious or chronic nature, there is still every hope that with counseling, the use of better stress-management tools, or even just the passing of time, the issue will be resolved and the cortisol levels will return to normal.

Unfortunately, if the reason for the elevated cortisol levels is physiological, such as inflammation, then, until the inflammation is resolved, the insomnia will persist. We are then back to a vicious cycle in which the loss of sleep creates more stress, and, in some people, an increase in stress will result in intestinal inflammation, since cortisol inhibits the body's repair processes. To make matters worse, it is while you are sleeping that the normal maintenance and repair processes occur, so if you aren't sleeping, you can't rebuild tissue effectively.

Often, in an effort to resolve insomnia, people will decide to enlist the aid of alcohol, especially if they are already experiencing pain in their joints or muscles. This only adds more fuel to the fire because alcohol will further degrade the intestinal lining, put an additional burden on the liver, and, since alcohol is technically a stimulant, it will contribute to the inability to successfully sleep through the night. Similarly, using one of the "P.M." preparations of anti-inflammatory medications designed for nighttime use will also further irritate the intestinal tract.

Research in sleep patterns has revealed that rapid eye movement (REM) or deep sleep occurs best when cortisol is at a low concentration, and that wakefulness (stage I sleep or slow wave sleep [SWS]) is associated with an increase in plasma cortisol concentrations. In controlled experiments, the administration of cortisol significantly decreased REM sleep. Similarly, in student cadets who were exposed to prolonged physical stress, increased cortisol levels and a disruption of circadian rhythms were recorded.

Conversely, DHEA secretion, which has a circadian rhythm opposite that of cortisol, should gradually climb as day turns into night. As discussed earlier, prolonged elevations of cortisol eventually result in decreased production of DHEA. A research study has shown that the oral administration of 500 mg of DHEA in healthy young men resulted in a significant increase in the amount of REM sleep.

DEPRESSION

Well, if you are not depressed by all of this so far, let me show you why you could be. People with endogenous depression (meaning that it is coming from imbalances in the biochemistry of the brain) exhibit hyperactive hypothalamic-pituitary-adrenal activity that is manifested by an increased secretion of cortisol and thus show significantly higher morning and midnight salivary cortisol levels.

A disruption of circadian sleeping rhythm due to elevated midnight cortisol levels was found in people suffering from depression. There is a great deal of scientific literature that discusses the relationship between cortisol circadian rhythms and daily fluctuations in depression and normal states of mind. This goes a long way in explaining why you can feel pretty good during one part of the day, and then, for no apparent reason, your mood sinks and you are depressed. It also highlights the importance of the twenty-four-hour adrenal stress index salivary test to chart the cortisol circadian rhythm.

People with endogenous depression are prone to further hypersecretion of cortisol when faced with recurrent or new stressors, meaning that they handle stress poorly. So here we are again, with a bad situation getting worse, and if you are one of these people, you don't have a clue to what is happening. There is really nothing occurring in the peripheral (exogenous) factors of your life, such as your job, your relationship with your spouse, or your finances, that could account for you being so depressed, but you are.

In my clinical experience I have found that people will create almost any "reality" in an attempt to justify what they think or feel. It's when they decide to blame their spouse, kids, boss, coworkers, etc., in an effort to find some reason to explain their depression that serious problems can begin. It's called "looking for trouble." This, of course, will make the object of your blame react in ways that are bound to make you even more depressed, such as when you receive your divorce papers or pink slip.

There is yet another avenue in which intestinal-tract inflammation and cortisol imbalances cause depression, and it is related to serotonin production. Serotonin is one of the neurotransmitter chemicals that makes us happy and most antidepressant medications work by blocking the brain's ability to reabsorb serotonin away from the cells that affect our mood. The theory is that the more serotonin available to these brain cells, the less depressed you will be. While antidepressant drugs work for some people, this theory completely ignores the fact that the brain is responsible for synthesizing only 1 percent of the body's total serotonin production, while the other 99 percent is synthesized in the intestinal tract. As it turns out, 99 percent of *all* of the body's neurotransmitters are made in the intestinal tract, so it is easy to see how any number of brain chemical disorders can occur if the intestinal wall is degraded and unable to make these chemicals that are vital to proper brain function.

Just understanding that one possible cause of your depression is a hormonal imbalance that can be tested for and treated can be very liberating, and it will take a lot of pressure off you and those around you. This by no means discounts other causes of depression involving imbalances in brain chemistry or the fact that tragic circumstances can justifiably cause depression.

CHRONIC FATIGUE SYNDROME

This syndrome is characterized by persistent or relapsing debilitating fatigue for at least six months, in the absence of any other definable medical diagnosis. Chronic-fatigue-syndrome patients exhibit low cortisol levels and adrenal insufficiency, meaning that their adrenal glands can no longer respond normally to ACTH stimulation from the pituitary gland and are in the fatigue phase of adrenal-gland maladaptation.

Symptoms of patients suffering from chronic fatigue syndrome include depression, insomnia, low blood pressure, obesity, and the inability to cope with stress. The cortisol deficiency may also lead to impairment of the immune system, evidenced by an elevation in the concentration of certain antibodies in people with this syndrome.

OBESITY

Cortisol secretion has been linked to obesity and is attributed to accelerated cortisol-production rates. Obesity related to elevated levels of cortisol can occur in several different ways.

First, many people use food as a means of reacting to stress. This will be discussed more comprehensively in a later chapter on diet, but suffice it to say that certain foods represent emotional comfort for some people, and they will gravitate to those foods to achieve the desired emotional state. For example, if Hostess Twinkies remind you of a happy time in your childhood, you might use them to emotionally transport you away from your adult stresses.

If you perceive your day as being stressful, you will most likely seek some way to reward yourself. Cortisol stimulates the area of the brain associated with the sense of being rewarded. At first, this may seem confusing, because why would we want cortisol to ring the bells in our brain's reward center? The apparent answer to this is that surviving a stressful event *is* rewarding and represents a desirable level of achievement. The time you might decide to reward yourself with food can occur during the day, while you are battling the slings and arrows of outrageous fortune or, more commonly, during the evening, when you are tired, at home, and have greater access to food.

Next, it is a fact that cortisol disturbs normal blood-sugar levels due to its effect on insulin, and this can easily cause a craving for sugar or carbohydrate-laden foods. The overconsumption of carbohydrates is an excellent way to gain weight because whatever glucose your body can't use will be stored as fat. If you exercise a lot, you will be able to exhaust the glucose stored in your muscles to the extent that you will convert the fat cells back to glucose as you continue to exercise. However, if you don't exercise enough to accomplish this, or if your imbalanced cortisol levels are also causing insomnia or chronic fatigue syndrome and you are too tired to exercise, cells are going to continue to accumulate.

There is also a relationship between cortisol and DHEA ratios in obesity. The administration of DHEA has been shown to have an anti-obesity effect in mice and rats: It causes a decrease in fat tissue and food intake.

IMMUNE-SYSTEM DISORDERS

As with obesity, both cortisol and DHEA levels have a dramatic effect on the immune system. In an experiment designed to measure the effect of cortisol on the body's production of white blood cells (T-lymphocytes) by challenging it with tetanus toxins, the oral administration of cortisol resulted in a 38 percent reduction of T-cell proliferation. These white blood cells also serve as regulatory and effector elements in *all* antigen-specific responses (antigens being defined as any substances that can elicit an immune response). These particular white blood cells also play a significant role in the immune system by interacting with other immune-system cells that eat up antigens.

As we discussed in Chapter 2, the reason cortisol is so highly immunosuppressive is because your body doesn't need an immune system under the circumstances of fight-or-flight stress, where the only agenda is survival. No doubt you may need your immune system after you have successfully fought off a predator and need to heal wounds you may have acquired, but while you are stressed, cortisol will suppress your immune-cell production. All of this is great for short-term stress, but it can be disastrous for long-term stress.

The T-cells are produced in the bone marrow and mature in the thymus gland, and DHEA protects the thymus gland from the effects of cortisol, which is just another example of how the body has a miraculous system of checks and balances to achieve homeostasis. It also helps to explain why every person who is stressed doesn't necessarily get sick. The immune system gets into trouble when the stress becomes chronic; the adrenal glands then go into maladaptive phases; and the cortisol/DHEA ratios become compromised. It is when the immune system becomes chronically imbalanced that the stage is set for an autoimmune disease.

In any autoimmune disease, the immune system can no longer distinguish which cells belong to the body and which don't, and it begins to attack them as if they were foreign cells, or antigens. An example of how the cortisol/DHEA ratio participates in autoimmune disease is rheumatoid arthritis.

Rheumatoid arthritis is an autoimmune disease that can cause inflammation of the joints throughout the entire body. It affects approximately 2 million Americans and is considered to be a chronic disorder. It begins when the immune system attacks the synovial membrane between the joints that produces the lubrication that allows the joints to glide smoothly. As the inflammation progresses, the joint becomes swollen and painful. Eventually, the cartilage lining of the joint is destroyed, and the pain increases. People with rheumatoid arthritis also exhibit low serum-DHEA levels.

IRRITABLE-BOWEL SYNDROME, ULCERS, AND COLITIS

One of the features of the human stress response, and the shift into the sympathetic nervous system mode that initiates it, is the shutting down of the parasympathetic nervous system that is responsible for digestion. This makes a great deal of sense because you need all of your blood to go to the muscles that can save you rather than to the organs contending with a Whopper and fries. This is bound to create problems if the stress becomes prolonged, the two most obvious of which involve hydrochloric acid production and mucosal lining repair.

One of the pioneers of the physiology of stress was Hans Selye, who in the 1930s performed experiments on rats involving ovarian hormonal extracts. In one of the great ironies of science, Selye was a seriously clumsy individual who had difficultly injecting the rats because he kept dropping them. In the interest of science, he had to chase and retrieve them in order to continue his experiments, and this proved to be a continuously stressful experience for the rats.

By the time he finished his experiment, he found that not only did the rats he injected with hormonal extracts have serious problems, but the ones he injected with saltwater only were also ill. As it turned out, both sets of rats had ulcers, debilitated immune systems, and enlarged adrenal glands. He thereafter embarked on a career of illustrating the effects of stress on physiology, which was the fortunate (for him, not the rats) result of his ineptitude in handling rats and scaring the hell out of them.

The reason the rats had so many ulcers is the fact that a part of the stress response is to shut down the body's repair mechanisms, which includes the mucosal lining of the digestive tract.

The enzymes that our bodies produce to break down the multitude of things, sometimes bizarre things, that we put into our stomachs are very powerful. Hydrochloric acid, pepsin, and bile are strong chemicals that our bodies require to deconstruct globs of proteins, carbohydrates, and fats. Since this is typically a three-times-a-day process, there is a continuous need for the body to repair the mucosal lining that protects the gastrointestinal tract from these caustic enzymes. However, mucus secretion is inhibited when cortisol levels are elevated.

Being stressed out doesn't mean you stop eating; in fact, as we have seen, some people eat more when they are stressed. This constant onslaught of food and enzymatic activity in the absence of repairing the mucosal lining will result in patches of irritation and inflammation. As we all know by now, one of the body's responses to inflammation is to produce more cortisol; so around and around we go. If this cycle continues, the tissues can be degraded until an ulcer or hole develops.

Activation of the sympathetic nervous system, which is the part of the nervous system that is activated in times of stress, will inhibit activity in the small intestines, where we absorb dietary nutrients, but will increase contractions in the large intestine, where waste products are processed and removed. The latter effect on the large intestine accounts for the phenomenon of literally having the poop scared out of you at times of extreme perceived danger.

Chronic hyperstimulation of the large intestinal tract from stress will result in irritation and diarrhea, and there are numerous medical diagnoses for these disorders ranging from colitis, irritable-bowel syndrome, and spastic colon, to diverticulitis. As is the case with the stomach and small intestinal tract, ulceration and bleeding can occur.

As a last thought regarding the effects of stress on the digestive tract, it is interesting to speculate on just what levels of dietary nutrients are actually being absorbed in people who are chronically stressed. Because it is in the small intestines where finger-shaped villi suck up nutrients and intestinal activity can be shut down during times of stress, it logically follows that chronically stressed people are unable to fully access food nutrients, which only adds to their feeling unwell and contributes to their susceptibility to illness. Of equal importance, in a chronically inflamed intestinal tract, the villi may be damaged or even disappear as the intestinal lining is damaged. This is an overlooked but very important aspect of human nutrition, because it is not only what you eat, but also what you actually absorb into your bloodstream that matters. The best diet in the world isn't going to do you much good if the nutrients are literally going in one end and coming out the other without being broken down and absorbed.

When I was in my first year of practice, I encountered a middle-aged man who was having an acute case of lower-back pain related to bending and lifting. I took an X ray of his lower spine, and to my horror I saw three areas of abnormal bone density over the outside of his pelvic bone that looked a lot like cancer to me. I wanted to be absolutely certain of the diagnosis and didn't want to alarm him by prematurely mentioning the possibility of cancer, so I called up a radiologist at the local hospital for a consultation.

I was rather nervous when he put the X ray on the light box because I was anticipating how terrible it was going to be to inform a patient that he had cancer. The radiologist looked at the film for several moments and burst out laughing. He informed me that while it was very reasonable for me to think that the white, dense shadows over the pelvic bone might be cancerous lesions, they were, in fact, calcium supplements that were passing through the intestinal tract completely undigested. At the time I took the X ray, the calcium tablets were making their way down the descending colon, which lies in front of the pelvic bone.

At that early point in my career, I was so happy that I didn't have to tell this guy he had cancer that I totally missed the relevance of *why* he wasn't digesting his calcium supplements. What had happened was that his stress levels were so chronically elevated from the stress of his job and personal life, along with the more recent stress of intense back pain, that his intestinal tract had slowed down to the point where he could not properly digest what he was eating.

What I now know is that no diet or vitamin supplement program is going to truly help any of the conditions I have been discussing in this chapter if you have an inflamed, debilitated intestinal tract or systemic inflammation that remains unresolved. For many people who suffer from chronic stress syndrome, intestinal tract inflammation may be the single most important issue to resolve, because if it persists, the cortisol and/or DHEA levels will remain imbalanced and perpetuate the digestive dysfunction. This results in the double whammy of having a digestive tract that has damaged or insufficient numbers of villi for absorption of nutrients and that is working at a pace that is too slow to produce the proper enzymes for digestion. Consequently, you will not be able to derive much benefit from the foods or vitamins that are necessary for good health.

OSTEOPOROSIS AND THYROID DISORDERS

These problems can be discussed together because both are the result of one hormonal imbalance causing another one.

The suppression of thyroid function caused by elevated levels of cortisol leads to hypothyroidism (low thyroid function) and related illnesses. In such cases, there are decreased serum-DHEA levels as well. The thyroid operates via a negative feedback loop in which the pituitary gland secretes thyroid-stimulating hormone (TSH), which causes the thyroid gland to produce triiodothyronine (T3) and thyroxin (T4). When the T3 and T4 hormones become appropriately elevated, the pituitary gland stops secreting TSH. Elevated levels of cortisol can block the normal sequence of how these hormones are made, which is why on abnormal thyroid tests, for example, the T3 may be too high while the T4 is too low or vice versa.

Another fascinating feature of thyroid imbalance, usually found in hypothyroidism, is that 20 percent of thyroid hormone conversion occurs in the intestinal tract, meaning that after the thyroid gland secretes hormones (T3), some of it has to be activated in the intestinal wall for it to become usable. If the intestinal tract is inflamed and compromised in its ability to function, this activation of thyroid hormone may not occur and for all intents and purposes, 20 percent of thyroid hormone is lost.

The symptoms of hypothyroidism are fatigue, low blood sugar, chronic infections, obesity (are you beginning to see a pattern here regarding the effects of cortisol imbalance?), intolerance to cold, muscle weakness, and constipation. Increased cortisol levels are also associated with osteoporosis in women and are linked to calcium malabsorption. An example of this syndrome is sometimes seen in elite female athletes with high levels of cortisol and exercise-related absence of menstrual cycles who exhibit significantly low bone-mineral density. Postmenopausal women with osteoporosis also show a low serum DHEA level and abnormal cortisol/DHEA ratios.

FIBROMYALGIA

Fibromyalgia is a disorder that began to gain notoriety in the mid-1980s and was initially viewed with scorn by the mainstream medical establishment because of its multiple symptomatology. As with chronic fatigue syndrome, it was given no credence, and people suffering with it were considered to be psychosomatic whiners with "yuppie flu." While no one seems to know what causes fibromyalgia, it is now taken seriously as an arthritis-related disease.

The symptoms of fibromyalgia are:

- Pain, which is usually widespread throughout the body in muscles, tendons, and joints
- Insomnia and fatigue
- Depression
- Anxiety
- Irritable bowel syndrome
- Difficulty with memory and concentration

The onset of fibromyalgia seems to correlate with an injury that has not been resolved and is causing chronic pain and/or elevated stress levels. Since this is the only disorder in this book for which I couldn't find a published research paper linking it to imbalanced cortisol levels, I am going to go out on a limb here and make the ever-popular "duck diagnosis": If it walks like a duck, looks like a duck, and quacks like a duck, then it probably is a duck. Given the extensive number of disorders in which I have shown cortisol involvement, and given the fact that these same problems occur together in fibromyalgia, it is probable that this is another form of an autoimmune disease precipitated by adrenal-gland imbalance.

It is my clinical opinion that if you have been diagnosed with fibromyalgia, then you are seriously in need of an adrenal stress index test to evaluate your cortisol levels and the status of your hypothalamic feedback loop. Even if imbalanced cortisol/DHEA levels are not the cause of fibromyalgia, it is quite logical to assume that just the stress and pain of this disease will upset the adrenal glands and ultimately result in hormonal maladaptation, and it is also logical that any effort to treat fibromyalgia should include rebalancing the cortisol/DHEA ratios if the saliva test proves there is an imbalance.

So far we have journeyed down a road of stress, disease, and despair, where adrenal-gland hormone imbalances and inflammation interact and can result in one health problem after another. Now it's time to explore how to get out of this mess, resolve your pain syndromes and inflammation, and correct your hormonal imbalances, so you can hopefully live happily ever after.

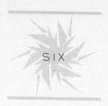

SIX

RESOLVING CORTISOL IMBALANCES

A Plan That's Easy to Follow and Swallow

The process of resolving cortisol imbalances requires an understanding of what *factors* are causing the imbalance and then the adoption of a logical "ladder" approach in correcting them. With the ladder approach, you start with the most obvious nutritional supplements that usually resolve the imbalance and then move step by step up the ladder if the first approach doesn't yield the expected results. Because hormonal function and balance are extremely complicated, something that works wonderfully for one person may not work as well for another.

This is why the adrenal stress index (ASI) test becomes so valuable, because it enables the doctor to assess what phase of maladaptation the adrenal glands are in, whether intestinal-tract inflammation is a factor, and whether the hypothalamus-pituitary feedback loop is functional. If the ASI indicates that an immune factor (SigA) of the intestinal tract is depressed or that gliadin antibodies to grain glutens (wheat, rye, oat, and barley) are elevated, then intestinal-tract inflammation is most likely present. After seeing the results of the ASI, your doctor may choose to order further tests to determine if you have *Candida albicans* or other bacterial or viral infection, and if the latter, he or she can order a C-reactive protein (CRP) test to determine the degree of inflammation. Once the results of the ASI are matched to the patient's symptoms, a nutritional supplement program can be initiated.

RELEVANT SYMPTOMS OF CORTISOL IMBALANCE

- Do you have trouble falling asleep? This problem usually indicates low blood sugar due to cortisol suppression of insulin. Or do you wake up in the middle of the night and have trouble falling back to sleep? This sleep disturbance is due to an abnormal elevation of cortisol, which causes alertness.

- Do you get depressed, angry, or anxious easily without reasonable provocation (the house hasn't burned down, you didn't lose your job, no loved ones are ill or have died, all of your retirement plan is not invested in Florida swamp land). This moodiness indicates that the adrenals are hyperfunctioning.

- Do you crave sugar? The suppression of insulin and interference with carbohydrate metabolism, caused by cortisol leads to cravings for sugar. Do you crave salt? Salt cravings are the result of a weakness in the adrenal glands' ability to manage the sodium-potassium pump that maintains the body's mineral content and the leakage of sodium out of the body. Do you crave chocolate? This is also a sodium-potassium pump problem, but it is magnesium that is leaking out, and chocolate is very high in magnesium.

- Are you tired all or most of the time, and do normal activities seem like too much of an effort to either start or finish? This lack of vitality would be caused by adrenal hypofunction and insufficient cortisol and DHEA.

- Are you a man, and your sex life can be described by the term *down and out*? Or are you a woman, and your attitude toward sex can be best described by "not *that* again?" This weak libido can be due to either adrenal hyper- or hypofunction, and the ASI will reveal the problem.

- Is your energy level generally good for the first part of the day but you fall into a slump either after lunch or around three or four o'clock in the afternoon? This fluctuation is the result of insulin resistance, which occurs when cortisol inhibits glucose from entering cells, the outcome being low energy and fatigue.

- Does your appetite seem relatively normal for most of the day until you eat dinner, after which you obsessively eat anything you can get your hands on? This is another example of an unbalanced relationship between cortisol and glucose levels.

- Do your hands and feet, or perhaps your entire body, feel cold most of the time even if the outside temperature is warm, or are you gaining weight even though you are not overeating? This would be indicative of a decrease in thyroid function that may be related to either adrenal and/or pituitary dysfunction.

Factors in Assessing the Risk of Intestinal-Tract Inflammation

- Have you ever taken or do you still take NSAIDs frequently? In a similar vein, have you taken prednisone or any other cortisone drug for a prolonged period of time?

- Have you ever been on long-term antibiotic therapy, even as long ago as your childhood ear infections?

- Do you consume caffeinated beverages, and if so, which ones (coffee, tea, soda), in what quantities, and how frequently?

- Do you drink alcohol, and if so, what type, in what quantities, and how often?

- Do you frequently experience intestinal bloating after eating, have a lot of flatulence, or feel like you have trouble digesting your food?

- Do you have either constipation or diarrhea frequently, or alternate between the two?

By piecing together the factors of cortisol imbalances as indicated by your symptoms with the results of the ASI, your doctor should be able to start you on the road to recovery. Again, it is important to remember that the hormonal system is exquisitely complex, and sometimes the nutritional supplements that work for one person will not always have the same effect on another.

THE CRITICAL IMPORTANCE OF HEALTHY RECEPTOR SITES

The receptor sites on cell membranes provide a perfect example of just how challenging the hormonal system can be. Remember, every cell in the body has receptor sites on its outer membrane wall, and these receptor sites are like little keyholes that are specific for particular chemical keys that attach themselves to the sites. These chemical keys can be nutrients, neurotransmitters, or hormones, and via this mechanism, the cell is able to selectively decide which chemicals go in and which go out, and what enzyme functions will occur. The *number* of receptor sites specific for hormones changes not only from day to day, but minute by minute! Obviously, for hormones to work properly, there must be an adequate number of receptor sites available, and if these sites are compromised for any reason, then hormonal function will be equally compromised. This may be one explanation for why one person who has a good number of receptor sites will improve more rapidly than another person whose receptor sites are diminished.

As we have seen in previous chapters, a major factor in receptor-site function is *plasticity*, which refers to the fluidity of the lipid (fat) membrane of the outer wall of each cell. The receptor sites are made of protein and are embedded in the lipoprotein membrane, and it is the plasticity or softness of the lipid wall that determines the sensitivity, function, and number of receptor sites. Diets that are high in trans-fats and omega-6 oils (most processed foods and certainly fast/junk foods) cause the lipid membrane to become stiff and reduce receptor-site function, whereas diets that are high in omega-3 oils promote membrane plasticity. This again points to the importance of diet in resolving cortisol imbalances far beyond the obvious affects of caffeine and sugar, because if the receptor sites are not able to adequately bind neurotransmitters and hormones, the cell cannot function at its optimal level.

Resolving Intestinal-Tract Inflammation: L-Glutamine

If the ASI test reveals that there is intestinal-tract inflammation, then treatment *must* begin with resolving the inflammation. It cannot be overstated how important this is, because no other therapy will have a meaningful long-term effect if the inflammation isn't addressed. You can take all manner of adrenal supplements or prescription Diflucan or nystatin for Candida infections, but unresolved intestinal inflammation will still cause the adrenal glands to produce cortisol as an anti-inflammatory hormone, and you will eventually enter the vicious cycle of inflammation-causing increased cortisol production, which will cause continued inflammation. As an analogy, consider a patch of weed-infested ground. You spray it heavily with weed killer, but then neglect to restore the area with healthy plants that would discourage the return of the weeds. Given just a little time, the weeds are going to grow back (as will the Candida in an unrepaired intestinal tract), and you are back to where you started.

Fortunately, resolving intestinal-tract inflammation is the easiest part of the program, and it can usually be repaired in as little as four to six weeks by simply taking 1,500 mg of the amino acid glutamine twice a day on an empty stomach. L-glutamine is one of twenty amino acids our bodies use to make protein, and there is abundant research that proves that glutamine plays a role in muscle formation; liver, kidney, and immune system function; and antioxidant production. There are virtually no known side effects to taking L-glutamine, except for the rare occurrence of constipation if there is too little water and fiber in the diet.

Back in 1978, a pharmacologist at the National Institutes of Health named Herbert Windmueller discovered that glutamine was the major fuel utilized by the cells of the intestinal tract and that a depletion of glutamine resulted in cellular death. Since then, there have been numerous research studies that prove the effectiveness of L-glutamine in repairing the mucosal lining of the intestinal tract, restoring the normal epithelial junctures or barriers (the little pinholes that result in leaky-gut syndrome), and improving the intestinal immune factors.

One of the most important research studies regarding glutamine was published in 1976 by Japanese scientists who induced ulcers in rats by giving them NSAIDs (aspirin, in this case). Two groups of rats were given the same amount of aspirin, but one group was also given L-glutamine. The administration of glutamine *totally* prevented the occurrence of ulcers in the rats. I find it interesting and very disturbing that while glutamine is the most commonly used antiulcer drug in all of Asia, it is virtually unknown and unused in this country. And there are numerous prescription and over-the-counter medications used to treat ulcers in the United States that have several negative side effects. Remember, this is a nation that has 16,500 deaths a year from prescription NSAIDs due to intestinal-tract bleeding, and these deaths could, for the most part, be prevented by simply taking L-glutamine (I recommed 1,500 mg) approximately one hour prior to taking the NSAIDs.

L-glutamine must be taken on an empty stomach to be clinically useful because when you eat and digest protein, the amino acids compete for absorption, and it is therefore impossible to predict how much glutamine will be absorbed. By taking the glutamine without any other amino acids from food, we can be sure that the body will get a good clinical dose. An empty stomach means that you have not eaten any protein for ninety minutes. The easiest way to take glutamine is upon arising in the morning because your stomach is certainly empty at that time, and again when going to bed at night, on the presumption that it has been an hour and a half since you had dinner and you have not eaten any protein since dinner. This is as easy as placing the bottle of glutamine on the nightstand next to your bed so when you wake up and go to sleep, it's right there waiting for you. Alternatively, you can take the glutamine thirty minutes before you are going to eat a meal with protein, such as taking it when you get home from work if you are not going to eat for the next half an hour.

Glutamine is easy to find in any vitamin or health food store, where it is sold as L-glutamine (the "L" simply signifies its molecular structure). It is inexpensive and is available in capsules that usually contain 500 mg of L-glutamine, so a 1,500-mg dose would mean three capsules. While I have seen several research articles that discuss much larger doses, in my clinical experience 1,500 mg twice a day is almost always enough to repair the intestinal tract in four to six weeks, as long as the patient is not taking NSAIDs, drinking a lot of caffeine (more than two 6-ounce cups a day), drinking a lot of alcohol (more than two drinks a day), or drinking sodas that contain phosphoric acid (zero a day because soda is garbage, plain and simple). And if the patient is mixing all of these factors together so that there are two cups of coffee, two sodas, two alcoholic beverages, and a couple of NSAIDs thrown in on a daily basis, forget about it! Basically, I ask my patients to decide which one of their vices is most important to them, to choose which ones they will give up in order to get well, unless they are so seriously ill that there is no room for compromise.

OTHER NUTRITIONAL SUPPLEMENTS FOR INTESTINAL-TRACT REPAIR

Glucosamine Sulfate

This is an amino sugar that is the progenitor of the building blocks of glycosaminoglycans, which are the key elements of connective tissue and the basement membrane to which the intestinal mucosa is anchored. Many people are aware of using glucosamine sulfate to enhance cartilage repair, and when I first started using it in my practice for that purpose, I was confused as to why the joints of some patients responded to it more quickly than others. Then I read a research article that informed me that doctors in England were using glucosamine sulfate to repair intestinal-tract linings. I realized that the patients who were taking longer to show improvement in their joints also had intestinal-tract inflammation and that the glucosamine sulfate was repairing the inflammation first before being utilized to create more joint cartilage. This understanding came long before I made the connection between intestinal-tract inflammation and cortisol imbalances.

Glutathione

This is a combination of three amino acids (cysteine, glycine, and glutamate), and it is a very powerful scavenger antioxidant, which means that it neutalizes oxygen free radicals that can destroy healthy tissue. It also helps to inhibit the production of the pro-inflammatory cytokines that occur in intestinal-tract inflammation.

Gamma Oryzanol

This is another potent antioxidant made from rice that supports the integrity of the intestinal tract, which means that it helps balance pro-inflammatory stimuli and supports normal intestinal glandular function.

Tillandsia

This occurs as fibrous masses on oak, pine, and cypress trees and contains fiber, iron, phosphorus, calcium, magnesium, manganese, chlorophyll, beta carotene, and B vitamins. It also contains coumarin and resins believed to possess antimicrobial properties.

Jerusalem Artichoke

This provides a good source of fiber, which also promotes the growth of beneficial intestinal bacteria, especially bifidobacteria.

Cellulase

This microbial enzyme is effective in breaking down insoluble fiber to simple sugars that can be fermented to short-chain fatty acids that nourish the intestinal tract.

These nutritional supplements do not have to be taken separately because Biotics Research Corporation makes a product called IPS (intestinal permeability support) that contains L-glutamine along with the above-mentioned supplements. Another option is a supplement called LGS-ZYME made by Apex Energetics which also contains a combination of herbs that are designed to stimulate growth and repair of the intestinal tract. The resource guide at the end of this book will assist you in finding a doctor who is familiar with Biotics and Apex Energetics products, since they can be obtained only through doctors and not in vitamin or health food stores. There are several fine suppliers of nutritional supplements, but in my clinical experience, I have found the products from Biotics Research Corporation and Apex Energetics to be the most effective and the easiest for patients to take. If your doctor has another supplier of nutritional supplements that he prefers, by all means go ahead and use the ones he recommends.

Resolving Systemic Inflammation

As I'll discuss in Chapter 8, systemic inflammation, which refers to elevated levels of inflammatory chemicals circulating throughout the body, can best be controlled by avoiding hydrogenated oils, fast foods, fried foods, baked goods, and processed foods that contain omega-6 oils. From a supplemental perspective, omega-3 oil from fish significantly reduces inflammation and is widely available at vitamin stores.

Make sure it is a good-quality oil and preferably one whose label says that it is pharmaceutical grade. A good-quality omega-3 oil will be screened for mercury, pesticides, and other toxins, and its label should state that it has been so screened. There are no clear recommended dosages, but I think 1,000 to 4,000 mg a day is certainly very safe and effective.

NUTRITIONAL SUPPORT FOR THE ADRENAL GLANDS

Once the repair of the intestinal tract is under way, it is time to consider nutritional support for the adrenal glands. Once again, there is no way I can overemphasize the importance of resolving the intestinal-tract repair *first*. By neglecting to do so, all other attempts to rebalance the adrenal glands are doomed to failure because cortisol will still be produced in response to the inflammation until the adrenal glands finally burn out and go into the adrenal fatigue phase of hypofunction. This doesn't mean that every case of adrenal dysfunction has to be accompanied by intestinal-tract inflammation, but it is always wise to check for it before proceeding with supplements for hormonal support.

This brings us to the topic of glandular extracts, which are nutritional supplements made from specific animal organs, usually bovine. Glandular extracts were widely used by medical doctors at the beginning of the last century and were manufactured by pharmaceutical companies such as Eli Lilly and Upjohn as recently as the late 1960s. These days, many medical doctors have little regard for glandular extracts and consider them to be nothing more than "meat pills" (a matter that I will address shortly), but such a position disregards the medical history of glandular extracts.

In 1919, during an epidemic of flu virus, Dr. Lucke at Camp Zachary Taylor in New York found that out of 126 people who died from the virus, 106 exhibited damaged adrenal glands upon autopsy and that the damage was due to the strain on the adrenal glands of being so ill. During this epidemic adrenal glandular extracts were administered to several hundred infected people who exhibited less debilitating symptoms as well as dramatically reduced periods of recovery.

Then, with the advent in the 1950s of antibiotics and cortisone (synthetic cortisol), medications developed to fight infection and inflammation, medical doctors simply turned away from glandular extracts and began prescribing mass quantities of these new wonder drugs (cortisone is three times more powerful than cortisol). Unfortunately, even when the significant negative side effects of cortisone became evident, medical doctors were sold on a drug that could only be obtained by prescription—and that generated windfall profits for the pharmaceutical company that manufactured it. And while there is no doubt that antibiotics have saved many thousands of lives, the overuse of these drugs has now created the problem of drug-resistant bacteria that can't be pharmaceutically killed, in addition to that of a significant percentage of the population that now has intestinal-tract inflammation.

So what are we to make of glandular extracts? Once ingested, aren't they burned up by the stomach's hydrochloric acid? Even if they are absorbed intact, how do they affect the specific organs they are intended for? Aren't glandular extracts really nothing more than dried "meat pills"?

In the References section, I provide the information necessary for you to find the sources that give all of the dry, scientific studies on glandular extracts, but what they boil down to is this: No, they are not simply dried "meat pills"; they are not burned up by the stomach's hydrochloric acid; they are easily absorbed intact by the digestive tract; and they do go directly to the target tissue and support that tissue's function. By example, the research proves that orally ingested thymus glandular extract makes its way to the thymus gland and improves the production, maturation, and activation of immune-system T-cells. And because glandular extracts can specifically reach the target tissue (e.g., adrenal, hypothalamus, pituitary), they are highly beneficial to the nutritional restoration of the corresponding gland. By correlating the results of the ASI with the patient's symptoms, a nutritional supplement program can be designed to meet the specific needs of each person.

When the ASI shows that the cortisol level is too low in any phase of the test, particularly if the adrenal glands are in a state of fatigue, then supplementation with adrenal glandular extracts is appropriate in restoring adrenal health. The dosage will vary, depending on how depleted the adrenal glands are and the quality of the glandular extract being used, and a doctor who is well versed in using these extracts will be your best resource. For those patients who do not wish to use glandular products, an herbal supplement called AdrenaStim is an easy-to-use skin cream made by Apex Energetics for adrenal fatigue.

The adrenal supplementation program does not always require glandular extracts, particularly in the case of vegetarians, and in fact, sometimes they are simply not appropriate in treating cortisol imbalances. Adrenal glandular extracts can elevate cortisol levels, and taking them obviously isn't going to resolve a cortisol imbalance if the cortisol is already too high. In this case we would use a supplement called ADHS (Biotics) or Adaptocrine (Apex Energetics), which lower or stabilize cortisol levels. ADHS and Adaptocrine contain a balance of vitamins and Chinese and Ayurvedic herbs that nutritionally support normal cortisol and DHEA levels. Keeping in mind that the ASI measures the cortisol levels four times throughout the day, (7:00 to 8:00 A.M., 11:00 A.M. to 12:00 P.M., 4:00 to 5:00 P.M., 11:00 P.M. to 12:00 A.M.), the supplement program can easily be tailored to the specific fluctuations in cortisol levels.

The point is, cortisol imbalances have lots of twists and turns, and it isn't as simple as the cortisol being either too low or too high. It can be normal during one part of the day, too low another part of the day, and then too high in another part of the day. This is the reason why it is important to treat each case on an individual basis and not to assume that the supplement program that works for one patient is going to yield similar results for the next patient.

DHEA

It is important in achieving-adrenal gland functional balance to maintain the proper cortisol/DHEA ratios, which will be a part of the ASI results. If the cortisol levels and the DHEA levels are too low, then it might be appropriate to take a DHEA supplement. It should be noted that no one should take DHEA if their cortisol levels are elevated because DHEA can be converted in the body to cortisol as well as to testosterone, estrogen, and progesterone. This is why you need to have your cortisol imbalances managed by a doctor who is experienced in this area and why you should not just run to the vitamin store every time you read an article that touts the next new fountain-of-youth supplement. If you are a woman who might be at risk for breast, uterine, or ovarian cancer, DHEA is definitely *not* a good idea.

Once again, the dosage of DHEA will vary, depending on the results of the ASI, but most of the time a dose between 25 and 50 mg is all that is required.

LIVER REPAIR AND DETOXIFICATION

There are other supplements that can be not only useful but necessary to fully repair all of the damage that can be caused by cortisol imbalances. Sometimes the liver becomes overburdened from the continual return of toxins that the intestinal wall is leaking out, in which case nutrients that support detoxification are needed. Another possible factor in liver toxicity is *xenobiotics,* which include plastics, organic solvents, pesticides, industrial wastes in water and air, and some medications. Most of the supplements that assist in liver detoxification are antioxidants that eliminate or neutralize free radicals. The appropriate nutritional supplements for liver detoxification are: glutathione, vitamins C and E, quercetin, magnesium, B-complex vitamins, copper, and zinc. Biotics makes a supplement called MCS (stands for Metabolic Clearing Support) and Apex Energetic makes one called Metacrin-DX that are both excellent for detoxifying the liver. Also, a really good-quality multiple vitamin/mineral complex will contain these nutrients and can be taken with no side effects. Milk thistle (sillymarin), an herb that is also very helpful in liver cleansing, can be found in most vitamin stores.

Killing the Candida Infection with Oregano Oil

Science is making rapid progress in unlocking Nature's basic secrets in plants and foodstuffs that provide more than just nutrients. One promising field of study is that of the variety of spices that have been used for centuries to add zest to a wide range of foods. And long before the advent of refrigeration it was recognized that herbs and spices could slow down food spoilage through natural antimicrobial activity. Recent studies have focused on the effects of spices and associated oils on food-borne organisms in the context of food safety and spoilage.

In the event the patient has an intestinal *Candida albicans* infection, I use sustained-release emulsified oregano oil, which can be very effective in eradicating the yeast. An analysis of oregano reveals that its oil contains two antioxidant compounds, thymol and carvacrol, that are effective in killing fungi and yeast. The Biotics Company makes a product called ADP, in which they have microemulsified the oregano oil, thereby dramatically increasing the effective surface area of the oil, and then applied a sustained-release mechanism. The combined effect of emulsification and sustained release is that it enhances the intestinal exposure to the oregano oil and its ability to eradicate the yeast.

Apex Energetics makes a supplement called MYCO-ZYME that also contains an extract of oregano oil and other herbal compounds for the removal of yeast and bacterial pathogens.

RESTORING THE HYPOTHALAMIC FEEDBACK LOOP WITH GLANDULAR EXTRACTS, PREGNENOLONE, AND PHOSPHATIDYLSERINE

When the hypothalamic/pituitary feedback loop has lost its sensitivity to cortisol, the end result is the oversecretion of ACTH by the pituitary gland, which, as you will recall, causes the adrenal glands to keep secreting more cortisol. In most cases, the hypothalamic/pituitary glands will respond well to glandular-extract supplementation, the dosage of which would obviously be related to each person's individual needs. If the glandular extracts do not effect the desired changes, or for vegetarians, there are two other viable approaches: pregnenolone and phosphatidylserine.

Pregnenolone is a hormone that is produced in both the brain and the adrenal glands, and like other steroid hormones, it is synthesized from cholesterol. Pregnenolone is considered a precursor hormone because it is essential to the synthesis of cortisol, DHEA, estrogen, and testosterone. When the ASI shows elevated levels of cortisol, especially in the late afternoon and evening, and decreased DHEA levels, it indicates increased ACTH stimulus from the pituitary gland. What is happening in this case is that pregnenolone is being diverted to making cortisol as opposed to making DHEA, a situation that will result in adrenal-gland imbalance. Nutritional supplementation of pregnenolone can cause an increase in DHEA and help regulate ACTH secretion. One of the advantages of supplementing with pregnenolone instead of DHEA is that the body can decide what to do with it, and it can help in other hormone imbalances that involve estrogen and testosterone. As is the case with DHEA, people need to be careful that they are not at high risk for reproductive-tract cancers, including prostate. Pregnenolone can be bought in vitamin and health food stores, but to proceed wisely, there should be an ASI test that indicates an actual need for it.

Phosphatidylserine has been shown to be very useful in optimizing hypothalamic/pituitary responsiveness and reducing the pituitary ACTH secretion that signals the adrenal glands to secrete cortisol. Phosphatidylserine is composed of lipids and phosphate and is mainly concentrated in brain cells, where supplementation has been noted to improve cognitive function and reduce depression.

A new and highly innovative form of phosphatidylserine is made by Apex Energetics and it is called AdrenaCalm, which instead of being in pill form is a cream that is applied to the skin. There are several advantages to having the delivery system of phosphatidylserine going through the skin, and they are related to effectiveness and cost. Very high doses are required for phosphatidylserine to be effective (up to 800 mg a day), which can translate into a lot of pills that are very expensive. The AdrenaCalm cream is inexpensive and allows hundreds of milligrams of phosphatidylserine to enter directly into the bloodstream which can rapidly lower cortisol levels, and in bypassing the digestive tract as it would in pill form, the phosphatidylserine avoids being broken down by digestive enzymes.

THE IMPORTANCE OF L-TYROSINE IN ADRENAL AND THYROID HORMONE PRODUCTION

The last nutritional supplement that can play a significant role in resolving cortisol imbalances is the amino acid L-tyrosine, which also can have a beneficial effect on thyroid and brain neurotransmitter function. In order for the adrenal glands and the thyroid gland to produce hormones, L-tyrosine must be adequately absorbed in the digestive tract from dietary protein. The adrenal glands convert L-tyrosine into epinephrine and norepinephrine in response to stress, and the thyroid gland combines L-tyrosine with iodine to make the hormone thyroxine, which regulates the body's temperature. L-tyrosine is also used by the nervous system to make the neurotransmitter dopamine, which relays nerve transmissions.

In my clinical experience, L-tyrosine can be enormously useful in patients who are in adrenal fatigue, those whose hands and feet (if not their whole bodies) are cold most of the time and who are easily depressed. I have seen the best results in cases that usually involve women who have a family history of thyroid problems and who often show only low-normal or even normal results on a thyroid blood test, even though they have the classic hypothyroid symptoms of fatigue, coldness, and depression. Often the patient shows an immediate improvement in all these symptoms after a week of tyrosine supplementation at a dosage of 500 mg twice a day on an empty stomach to ensure complete absorption.

L-tyrosine, however, is absolutely not for everybody, and it must be used carefully. L-tyrosine can raise blood pressure and should never be used in people who have hypertension, even if they have hypothyroid symptoms. For the same reason, L-tyrosine should not be used by those who are prone to vascular headaches or migraine headaches. Lastly, L-tyrosine should never be taken in conjunction with antidepressant drugs containing monoamine oxidase (MAO) inhibitors, as the blood pressure could elevate to very high levels.

CHROMIUM

Chromium is a trace mineral that has been found to be very effective in controlling sugar cravings since it affects insulin regulation. It can also be useful in lowering cholesterol levels, especially triglycerides, as elevated cholesterol is more a problem of carbohydrate management than fat consumption. Chromium is important in cases of insulin resistance (syndrome X) and, therefore, diabetes.

The most effective dosages I have found are 200 mcg twice a day. If you are taking the multiple vitamin/mineral supplements I recommend in Chapter 8, then you might be getting enough chromium. If not, chromium can easily be bought in a vitamin store, and this is one supplement that is very safe and that probably everyone should be taking.

Climbing Up the Ladder of Hormonal Balance

A concise review of the ladder approach to treating cortisol imbalances looks like this: First an adrenal stress index (ASI) test is completed by the patient and sent to the laboratory for analysis, then the doctor who ordered the test receives the results and uses them to establish a treatment protocol specific to the patient's needs.

- Presence of intestinal-tract inflammation indicated by low SigA, high C-reactive protein, or intestinal permeability tests = L-glutamine at 1,500 mg twice a day on an empty stomach or IPS (Biotics) or LSG-ZYME (Apex Energetics) two pills three times a day for four to six weeks.
- Any part of the day that the ASI indicates an elevated cortisol level = ADHS (Biotics) one to two pills, or 200 mg phosphatidylserine (AdrenaCalm by Apex Energetics) per day, used during the part of the day the cortisol is elevated.
- Any part of the day that the ASI indicates a decreased cortisol level = 80 to 160 mg per day of adrenal glandular extracts (Biotics), depending on ASI results, or Adaptocrine (Apex Energetics) two pills and/or AdrenaStim (Apex Energetics) cream during periods of decreased cortisol levels.
- ASI reveals a loss of hypothalamic pituitary sensitivity and ability to suppress ACTH secretion = 40 to 80 mg hypothalamus/pituitary extract (Biotics) a day or 200 mg phosphatidylserine (AdrenaCalm by Apex Energetics) a day at any part of the day when the ASI indicates an elevated cortisol level.
- ASI shows a low DHEA level = 10 to 25 mg DHEA morning and possibly afternoon, depending on results of test, or 25 mg pregnenolone once a day.
- ASI shows high gliadin antibodies or testing for *Candida albicans* is positive = ADP emulsified oregano (Biotics) or MYCO-

ZYME (Apex Energetics) two pills, three times a day for four to six weeks, or if it is a particularly severe case, medical intervention of nystatin or Diflucan may be necessary. Upon completing a treatment protocol for Candida or any other microbial infection of the intestinal tract, it is essential that a good-quality probiotic supplement containing *Lactobacillus acidophilus* and *Bifidobacterium bifidum* be taken for at least one month to restore the normal flora to the intestinal tract.

- Cases in which women have a family history of thyroid disorders, especially hypothyroid symptoms of fatigue, bodily coldness, and depression = 500 mg L-tyrosine twice a day on an empty stomach. In the event that the L-tyrosine does not resolve the thyroid symptoms, there are other excellent supplements that can be helpful, such as Thyro-Stim (Biotics) or Thyro-CNV (Apex Energetics), and your doctor will be able to advise you about this.

In most cases of cortisol imbalances, a positive response to therapy should be realized in as little as six weeks and certainly by three months. Your doctor may want to do a follow-up ASI test after two to three months, depending on your progress, and in other cases the progress is so obvious that the supplement program is commensurately reduced and then discontinued.

While the subtitle of this chapter is "A Plan That's Easy to Follow and Swallow," I realize that the above protocols may appear overwhelming. I want to reassure you, however, that hardly anyone except the most severe cases needs all that supplementation. For most people with cortisol imbalances, it's a short program that usually consists of L-glutamine and one or two glandular extracts to resolve the problem. It is also important to remember that in most cases, the program is intended to bring the body back to a state of balance or homeostasis, at which point further supplementation is not required.

The most typical exception to this is when the circumstances of a person's life are unalterably stressful, such as going through the chronic illness of a loved one. And even when this does occur, usually the supplementation program can be minimalized once the greater part of the imbalances are corrected.

No one, and I really mean *no one* reading this book should take the above information and run out to the health food or vitamin store and randomly start taking glandular extracts, DHEA, pregnenolone, tyrosine, or anything else, without first consulting a doctor qualified to assess your condition and personal need for *any* supplementation. One of the reasons for writing this book is not only to stress the dangers of cortisol imbalances, but to guide you toward proper diagnosis and treatment, which occur far too infrequently. One of the legitimate complaints that traditional medicine has regarding vitamin and nutritional supplementation is that there is a lot of misinformation out there, and there are slapdash "therapies" that have no basis in science or even reason. Unfortunately, people waste a lot of money chasing magic-bullet "cures" that don't work, and they simply don't get better and have a better quality of life.

Just as many movies or commercials that contain dangerous stunts advise "Do not attempt this at home," I am imploring you to use the resource guide at the end of this book in order to find a local doctor or acupuncturist who can order and evaluate these tests for you, follow through with the appropriate program, and help you *get well!*

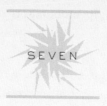

SEVEN

MAKE THE PAIN
GO AWAY

Treating *Causes* Instead of *Symptoms*

Chronic pain usually results in long-term use of NSAIDs (nonsteroidal anti-inflamatory medications such as aspirin and ibuprofen), which, as we have seen, eventually leads to intestinal inflammation and leaky-gut syndrome, which in turn leads to cortisol imbalances and a host of other problems. It is obviously important to try to resolve the *cause* of the pain rather than continue to merely treat the symptoms. Referring back to the components of the triangle of health, if a structural component is compromised, thereby causing pain and stress to the body, then the pain must be resolved in order to keep cortisol levels balanced.

Pain in America, a report prepared by the Merck pharmaceutical company in March 2000 and presented to the American Arthritis Foundation, stated the following: "Eighty-nine percent of the people polled reported having some sort of pain on a monthly basis; 68 percent experienced pain weekly; and 42 percent reported having pain daily. Of those who had pain daily, 23 percent reported joint pain; 22 percent reported back pain; 18 percent reported arthritis; 13 percent reported headaches; and 12 percent reported neck pain." Remarkably, 65 percent of these people believed that stress was a factor in their pain syndromes.

Over the years, there has been so much misinformation regarding the cause of and appropriate treatment for joint pain, whether it's back, neck, or other joints, that it has made it very difficult for patients to decide what type of therapy is best for their condition. Fortunately, from years of extensive research, there is a compelling amount of evidence supporting the positive effects of spinal and joint manipulation. One of the most comprehensive research studies comes from the U.S. Department of Health and its Agency for Health Care Policy and Research (AHCPR), which was established to determine what are the most effective forms of treatment for specific disorders. In December 1994, this multidisciplinary panel recommended spinal manipulation as a highly effective treatment for lower-back pain. Another research study done at Duke University in 2000 proved that spinal manipulation is very effective for treating headaches and ranked it as a superior form of treatment when compaired to prescription drugs, over-the-counter drugs, and acupuncture. These studies did not specifically use the term *chiropractic,* but the reality is that with the exception of some osteopaths, chiropractors are the only doctors specifically trained and qualified to perform spinal and joint manipulation.

Chiropractic care has several different adjusting techniques for performing spinal manipulation, most of which are extremely gentle. The perception that chiropractic adjustments resemble something out of World Federation Wrestling is grossly erroneous. There are methods of spinal manipulation or adjusting that utilize a handheld instrument that delivers a precisely measured thrust to the joint; other times a gentle thrust of the thumb is all that is needed; and sometimes simply having the patient lie on strategically placed cushioned wedges that adjust the pelvic girdle is all that is required. These methods are also ideal for adjusting other joints, such as shoulders, knees, and elbows. The Resource Guide at the end of the book will help direct you to doctors who perform these techniques.

WHERE THE PAIN IS COMING FROM

Since its inception in 1895, chiropractic philosophy has embraced the concept that the nerves exiting the spinal cord between the vertebrae control most of the body's functions and that the ability of these spinal nerves to properly transmit messages between the brain and the rest of the body can become altered or compromised if there is a dysfunction in vertebral joint mechanics. The belief was that the spinal nerves were being pinched or compressed, which would alter their ability to function normally. While this phenomenon does occur and does cause pain, which is more likely to radiate down an arm or a leg, it is not the sole reason for joint pain.

Fortunately, with recent advances in neuroscience, it is now understood that the primary basis for joint pain involves the nerve cells that are actually inside the joints. These cells, called *mechanoreceptors,* are concerned with the mechanical function of the joint as well as with *proprioception,* or balance.

In numerous studies involving automobile whiplash injuries, researchers have concluded that the damage responsible for eliciting pain has occurred to either the spinal joints and/or the discs between the vertebrae, and that both of these structures are loaded with mechanoreceptor nerve cells. In this type of injury, the joint's ability to move in its normal functional range has been compromised by the traumatic impact, which results in the *understimulation* of mechanoreceptor stimuli. Essentially, the joint is stuck in a position that doesn't allow for adequate mechanoreceptor stimulation, which is also the case in lifting injuries, sports injuries, and even sleeping in the wrong position. If enough of the mechanoreceptors in any given joint are sufficiently understimulated, it activates or turns on the mechanoreceptor pain fibers, which fire pain stimuli to the brain. Damage to the discs also results in poor mechanoreceptor innervation and pain. This is a major reason most people with spinal or other types of joint pain find that they are often in more pain in the morning after they have been lying still for six to eight hours and improve somewhat after moving around, in effect, getting their mechanoreceptors restimulated.

Another interesting facet to this is how so many people with joint pain swear they feel better after a hot morning shower, which leads them to believe that heat is beneficial to their condition. The reality is that the only other place in the human body that has mechano-receptor nerve cells is the skin. What is actually happening is that the water from the shower head is stimulating the skin and the mechano-receptors, and any time you stimulate the mechanoreceptors, the pain will abate. The reason manipulation of spinal and other joints, as performed by chiropractors and osteopaths, relieves pain is that it restores the joint to its normal range of motion and enables the mechanore-ceptors to regain normal stimulation.

How It's All Wired Together

There is an enormous neurological consequence to mechanorecptor dysfunction, which is related to how these cells are wired into the spinal cord. Mechanoreceptors synapse or fire into a place called the *seventh lamina* (layer) of the spinal cord, which is also where we find the nerve fibers that go to muscles, the immune system, the vascular system, the adrenal glands, and most other organs. Therefore, chiro-practors also believe that many health disorders, including those in-volving organ function, may have their basis in mechanoreceptor dysfunction that can benefit from spinal manipulation, which chiro-practors also call *spinal adjustments.*

An example of the far-reaching neurological effects of spinal manip-ulation can be found in a current research study that shows that spinal manipulation has the *direct result of decreasing cortisol secretion* and, there-fore, dramatically increases immune function. This is an ongoing study from Australia that began in 2002 and involves 420 patients with an average age of forty-six, in which the effects of spinal manipulation on asthma, depression, and anxiety were investigated. Other forms of manual therapy, such as massage, were also tested, but researchers found that only the group that received spinal manipulation displayed significant improvement in asthma symptoms, depression, and anxiety scores.

Chiropractic care takes into account the triangle of health and addresses its structural, chemical, and emotional components. As such, chiropractic care can consist of spinal and other joint manipulation; physiotherapy modalities, such as ultrasound; nutritional counseling; hormone testing and balancing programs; postural education; strengthening and stretching programs; and techniques for neuro-emotional stability.

If you have been suffering with a pain syndrome that simply will not resolve with medical care, or if the symptoms are only alleviated by taking medication that sooner or later is going to produce an unwanted side effect, then you are an excellent candidate for chiropractic care. The ultimate goal of chiropractic care is to treat the *cause* as opposed to the symptom, and since the nervous system is connected to nearly every one of your cells, it's not hard to understand that neurological imbalances can have far-reaching health consequences. If you don't find a way to resolve your pain, and the stress it inflicts on your body, it's hard to imagine how you will keep your cortisol levels balanced.

If you have tried everything from traditional medical care, chiropractic care, acupuncture, physical therapy to even witch doctors and *still* can't find relief, there are three factors that have probably been overlooked. These three factors are: psoas-muscle spasm, ligament instability, and a craniosacral syndrome.

The Importance of Psoas-Muscle Balance

One of the first things that can go wrong when a lower back, hip joint, shoulder, or neck problem won't resolve is that there is probably an undetected psoas-muscle spasm. The psoas muscles are two of the most important muscles in the lower back, one on each side.

They attach the ball of the hip to the socket of the pelvis; they are firmly attached to the front of all five of the lower-back vertebrae, including the discs; and they end at the last two vertebrae that have ribs attached to them (technically, the bottom of the shoulder girdle).

The psoas muscles are responsible for two functions. When they contract individually, they cause the knee to flex toward the waist as in walking, running, climbing stairs, or riding a bicycle. When both psoas muscles contract at the same time, you are either lying on your back pulling your knees up toward your chest or you are bending over at the waist. It is bending over at the waist that gets most people into trouble with their lower backs. Since lower back pain is a leading cause of people seeing a doctor, each day doctor's offices around the world are filled with patients who tell a tale of woe about how they injured their backs by lifting while bending or simply by reaching forward. In many cases they weren't even lifting something heavy, and the movement could have been as innocuous as putting on their socks.

What has happened is that their psoas muscles are already overly tight, and as they engage in forward bending activities, it becomes a case of the straw that breaks the camel's back: It's just one time too many. At that point they are so close to the muscle going into a full-scale spasm that it only takes a few more forward movements for the spasm to occur. Sometimes it can go into spasm as the end result of repetitive flexion activities, such as gardening or house cleaning.

When this occurs, patients often describe feeling as though their back "went out" or "gave way." What they are describing is the dramatic effect of one of the psoas muscles becoming so spastic that it pulls the lumbar spine and pelvic girdle into a fixated position that no longer enables it to function within its normal range of motion. As we have discussed, this results in the understimulation of the mechanoreceptor nerves and triggers the pain fibers. The pain can range from discomfort to complete debilitation, preventing the patient from standing up straight or walking properly.

People with chronic lower-back pain will frequently notice that the pain can travel upward and result in neck or shoulder pain. It is always interesting when, during a consultation with a new patient, they first tell me all about their history of lower-back pain and then at some later point they mention a shoulder problem they have acquired without incurring any injury or trauma. It never occurs to them that the two problems are related. Because the psoas muscles are attached to the bottom of the shoulder girdle, when one muscle goes into spasm, it will pull down on the shoulder and create an anatomical and physiological imbalance. It is hard to predict which shoulder will have pain, as it could be the one that is too low or the one that is too high. Similarly, it is just as difficult to predict which side of the lower back might be more painful relative to which psoas muscle has gone into spasm, and it is not unusual for the pain to be worse on the side opposite the muscle spasm.

Most certainly, not everyone with lower-back, hip, shoulder, or neck pain has a psoas-muscle involvement, but if you are the unlucky person who tends to incur this muscle imbalance, you are not going to achieve a level of continued stability if it's not corrected. Instead, you will be the person who fears the next episode of lower-back pain that you are sure is coming from some simple activity that requires bending over from the waist. The truly good news is that it takes exactly ten seconds to correct it, and you can do it lying in bed at home. And in my next book I am going to tell you how. Okay, okay, then! We'll take care of this now.

The technique for correcting a psoas-muscle spasm is so easy that most patients try to mess it up and make it more complicated than necessary. Since we can't be sure which muscle is involved without properly examining you, the next best thing is to do the corrective procedure on both sides, which is completely safe. The technique is identical for both sides, so while the instructions I am giving are for a right psoas-muscle spasm, obviously you would just reverse it to resolve the left psoas muscle.

1. Lie on your back in bed and bend your right knee up, keeping your right foot flat on the bed.

2. Place your left hand one inch to the right of your navel.

3. Press your left hand gently down into your abdomen and, while holding that pressure, slowly swing your right knee toward your left leg ten times, still keeping your right foot flat on the bed. This will feel like you are doing absolutely nothing of any benefit because most of the time it causes no pain or discomfort. If you are thinking nothing is happening, you are mistaken. I promise you that this simple procedure will resolve the psoas spasm.

4. Repeat this procedure on the left side.

There is a logic I impart to my patients when I teach them to do the psoas correction, which is that while it is very important that they get back into proper alignment, it is equally important that they *stay* that way. If I put a patient back in alignment and neglect to correct a psoas-muscle spasm, just how long should we expect that patient to stay in alignment considering that he is going to have to use his psoas muscle to walk out of my office? It is my guess that he will be lucky if he makes it to his car before the spastic psoas muscle begins to pull him off-center again.

These are the kinds of patients who will say they have trouble "holding" their adjustments, or they give up treatment because they don't stay well for very long. Or if it isn't their lower back that hurts then it's their neck, or their shoulders, or it's always something. They never achieve meaningful stability, and they also develop a well-deserved paranoia about their bodies because they feel they are walking time bombs; they never know which time they bend forward or reach for something that they are going to end up in pain. They grow wary of activities that used to be fun for fear of pain, and it limits the quality of their lives.

If you happen to be one of these unlucky souls, then your best defense is to do the psoas-muscle corrective procedure *every* morning before you get out of bed and *every* night when you get back into bed. You can also do it before and after an activity that will require some flexion, such as gardening. It is important to understand that you are trying to prevent a problem from occurring, so you should do this even if you are not experiencing pain. By example, you brush your teeth every day, not just when they hurt.

Since the psoas muscles are responsible for the ability to bend from the waist and that activity causes more lower-back pain than anything else, it is equally important that you learn to bend your knees to reach for things that are lower than you are. It is not just when lifting heavy objects that it is important, but it is the repetitive strain on the psoas muscles that gets a lot of us into trouble.

It takes human beings about thirty days to develop a new muscle memory pattern, and considering you have been bending over incorrectly for most of your life, you have to be patient with yourself in learning to bend with your knees. No doubt, after two weeks you will still catch yourself bending incorrectly, but if you persevere for the whole thirty days, you will get the hang of it. Ideally, you want to reach a point where you almost never bend over at the waist, and if you have to, you are still bending your knees to transfer the strain from your lower back to your thigh muscles.

If your spinal or other joints are fixated and not in normal alignment, however, doing the psoas corrective procedure alone will not put you back in alignment. You will still need to see a chiropractor or an osteopath who does manipulation if you are ever going to recover. The point is, if you are out of alignment and that is the cause of your pain or symptoms, you are not going to get better until you get back into alignment. You can put ice on it, use heat, do ultrasound, rub it, medicate it, and even perform surgery on it, but in the end you are still out of alignment and in a state of neurological dysfunction.

By no means should this be construed to mean that chiropractic or manipulative care is appropriate for every condition, and I can assure you that if you ever saw me carve a Thanksgiving turkey, you do not want me performing your appendectomy. Manipulative care is obviously not the treatment of choice for broken bones, cancers, or pathological or psychiatric diseases.

Achieving Ligament Stability

The second problem I most frequently notice when a person in pain has tried chiropractic or manipulative care and either has not recovered very well or has not achieved lasting stability, is that he or she has not been properly instructed on the importance of cold compress therapy.

Nearly everything that goes wrong with joints, ligaments, tendons, and muscles involves inflammation. From a medical perspective, this is why anti-inflammatory medications are prescribed. One of the major problems with this approach, aside from the intestinal-tract inflammation side effects described earlier, is that the medications don't work very well with respect to joint and ligament injuries. Joints and ligaments are by and large *avascular*, which means they have a minimal blood supply. This makes it difficult for a medication that is taken orally and delivered through the bloodstream to effectively reach these tissues.

As a chiropractor, I often reflect on the fact that if anti-inflammatory medications worked as well on joint and ligament problems as medical doctors and patients hoped, there wouldn't be as much need for chiropractic care. Instead, the single most common phenomenon in any chiropractic office is the new patient who has a history of using NSAIDs and is complaining about how the NSAIDs did not relieve his or her pain.

While the use of cold compresses is frequently recommended, especially in the acute phase of an injury or pain syndrome, the patient is usually not instructed properly as to how long to use them or even given the rationale for their use. When I see patients who have been told to use cold compresses but still do not get well, the reason is always the same: They were told to use the cold compresses only at the onset of pain and to use them only for the first three days. This fails in ways that are incredibly shortsighted.

First, the inflammation is definitely going to last more than three days. I find it very interesting that the same doctor who tells patients to use cold compresses for only three days will, at the same time, put them on a one-month prescription of NSAIDs. The application of cold compresses to resolve inflammation must be used on a consistent, long-term basis, often for as long as four to six weeks.

Second, and most important, ligaments are the tissues that hold the joints together, but they are the slowest-healing tissue in the body. If the ligaments don't fully heal and regain the tensile strength necessary to hold the joints in proper functional alignment, then a complete recovery may never occur, increasing the chance of reinjury. This would be a situation where the patient finds that every time he engages in strenuous activity he runs the risk of recurring pain because he is placing stress on ligaments that have never fully healed and are therefore unable to keep the joints stable. If you combine this problem of ligament instability with an undetected psoas-muscle spasm, it's easy to see how much trouble a person can get into with activities requiring bending forward. It is a generally accepted fact that ligaments take a minimum of four to six weeks to repair, although there is research that states it could take longer, depending on the degree of trauma involved.

Ligaments are composed primarily of collagen, whose molecules bind together in a cold environment, like the gelatin product Jell-O. While Jell-O has to be heated up on the stove to get all of the ingredients to combine evenly, it won't acquire that wobbly, gelatinous consistency until it's placed in the refrigerator. Gelatin products contain much less collagen than your ligaments do, which is a good thing, unless you want to be Gumby or a contortionist. By using cold compresses on a joint or ligament injury for the entire four to six weeks required to heal the ligaments, you are giving them the opportunity to fully bind together and regain their normal tensile strength.

Another reason for using cold compresses on areas where ligaments are subjected to stress is the prevention of injuries. My favorite story about this subject involves a forty-two-year-old male in the concrete-pouring business who came to see me with a history of chronic lower-back pain. He went through a typical course of treatment, became completely pain free, and was released from further treatment. My parting advice to him was that if he wanted to reduce the risk of another injury, he should use cold compresses on his lower back every day that he worked in order to prevent the ligaments from becoming progressively weakened.

I have given this advice over and over again for many years and frankly, hardly anyone listens. The reason for this is the brain's ability to forget pain, and without the pain to remind us, we simply stop doing the things that would prevent it.

About two and a half years later this patient returned to my office for care. Being a creature of presumption, I asked what was wrong with his lower back. He surprised me by saying that his lower back was fine, but he had slept on his stomach and woken up with neck pain. My curiosity regarding his lower back was no less diminished, and I asked him about it again since it had been such a long time between visits. He told me that he had actually used the cold compresses on his back every day after work, and the pain had never returned.

The point here is that the use of cold compresses can be preventative as well as curative. Unfortunately, most of us have been raised by mothers who dragged out the heating pad for every ache and pain, and we have a measure of doubt about using cold because it sounds like it may be uncomfortable. In reality, the cold is very soothing and brings an almost immediate sense of relief. However, for it to be effective, it must be used properly and with some common sense.

First of all, we are talking about cold compresses and not the direct application of ice on the skin. This can best be accomplished by using a soft gel pack, which can be found in most pharmacies, and putting it in the freezer until it gets cold. The trick of turning an ice pack into a cold pack involves nothing more than placing a towel between the pack and your skin. As people have different tolerances to cold, I advise my patients to put enough towels and/or clothing in between so that they are comfortable.

The cold compress should be applied for twenty minutes at a time and not any longer. It isn't a case of the longer you use it, the better the result you will get. However, it is true that the more frequently you use the cold compresses, the faster you will heal. For the average working person with the typically busy schedule, the best one can hope for is using the compresses twice a day: perhaps once before or after dinner and then again before bedtime. On days off or on weekends, the frequency of application could be increased. You should allow one hour between applications.

When Heat Can Help

There is a place for therapies that utilize heat, but most of the time it involves the types that will be found in either a doctor's or a physical therapist's office. Therapies such as ultrasound or short-wave diathermy have value because of their ability to penetrate from one to four inches into the body and alter the chemistry of the muscles. The old heating pad at home has very poor penetration capabilities and will not have much effect on the lactic acid content of a spastic muscle.

The primary value of using heat therapies on tight muscles is to remove lactic acid that can become congested in the muscle. Muscles utilize glucose for fuel and give off lactic acid as a waste product of this process. Under normal circumstances, once the muscle relaxes, the lactic acid gets dumped out into the circulatory system, where it is transported to the kidneys and excreted into the urine. However, if the muscles remain in a state of abnormal prolonged contraction due to an aberrant nerve supply, the lactic acid will become trapped inside and cause further problems.

For example, the patient is out of alignment, so the nerves going to a particular muscle group are overly excited and are causing the muscles to go into spasm. Unlike physical exercise, when the muscles relax once that activity ceases, the muscles receiving the excessive nerve signals remain in a state of contraction. Keep in mind that muscles only do what the nerves tell them to do. (The only exception to this is the presence of some other chemical imbalance in the muscle, such as a calcium deficiency, which is rare.) So now the chiropractor is trying to get the patient back into alignment, but the tight muscles are resisting and pulling the alignment out again.

While there is plenty of research that proves that spinal manipulation will cause muscles to relax, sometimes the muscle is so congested with lactic acid that the muscle rebounds and goes back into spasm. The problem is that if the concentration of lactic acid inside the muscle becomes too elevated, it will cause the muscle to contract further. The muscle becomes stuck in a cycle of abnormal nerve supply, causing a spasm and a buildup of lactic acid, which just perpetuates the condition. An excess of lactic acid is responsible for the burning type of pain people experience in their muscles. In the early days of aerobic dance classes, it was popular for the instructors to urge participants to "feel the burn." This fell out of fashion as it became apparent that the muscles were being overused and damaged.

Research on Olympic athletes shows that cold compresses disperse lactic acid from muscles as well as heat does, but in the case of prolonged spasms, there again is the problem of effectively penetrating the muscle. This is where ultrasound or short-wave diathermy can be useful by using sound or radio waves to push the heat deep into the muscle tissue, thereby dispersing the lactic acid. By clearing the lactic acid out, the muscle has a better chance of resuming its relaxed state while the nervous system is being normalized by spinal manipulation.

It is also worth mentioning that drinking sufficient amounts of water is essential to the body's elimination of lactic acid. If you find that you get stiff muscles easily with activity or exercise, then you are probably not drinking enough water, and you could be putting yourself at risk of an injury due to overly tight muscles.

Allowing for this brief discourse on heat therapies, cold compresses at home are still the best way to go for most pain syndromes, whether they are acute or chronic. As I stated before, the failure to use cold compresses properly constitutes the second factor in the list of problems that can prevent recovery from joint and ligament injuries.

CRANIOSACRAL THERAPY

The third factor that might account for a patient's failure to recover is that there is something wrong with his head, literally and structurally. In both the chiropractic and osteopathic professions there is a treatment known as *craniosacral therapy*.

The premise of craniosacral therapy deals with an aspect of human physiology known as the *primary respiratory mechanism,* which refers to the movement of cerebrospinal fluid from the brain down through the spinal cord. One of the most important features of craniosacral function is that a rhythmic motion occurs at the sutures where the bones of the skull meet and that there is a corresponding motion in the membranes covering the brain and the spinal cord. The sacral part refers to the last bony segment of the spinal column that people commonly call their tailbone, which also has a rhythmic motion that is synchronized with the cranial bones. Because the cerebrospinal fluid is the liquid medium that transports all of the oxygen and nutrients used by the brain and the spinal nerves, the ability of the cranial bones to move normally and assist in the flow of this fluid is vitally important.

The traditional-medicine community initially rejected this concept of cranial motion because according to accepted curricula, the sutures of the skull become fused by the age of twenty-five. The idea that these bones could move and, even worse, become misaligned and thereby adversely affect human health was met with great derision.

One of the first doctors to advance the concept of craniosacral motion was an osteopath named William Sutherland. In 1939, to prove that the sutures did not fuse together, he performed an experiment whose simplicity and brilliance you just have to love. Dr. Sutherland took the skull of a fresh cadaver, cleaned it out until all of the tissue was gone, and filled the inside of the skull with dried beans. He then placed the skull in a large pot of water and went to bed. Upon arising the next morning he found that the sutures of the skull had disarticulated and separated because of the expansion of the beans.

Of course, it was the medical community who thought Dr. Sutherland was the one full of beans, and craniosacral motion remained a controversial subject. In the end it was Dr. Sutherland who had the last laugh, although he did it in the confines of his grave, because researchers at Michigan State University College of Osteopathic Medicine have confirmed cranial motion using X-ray studies of living skulls.

Craniosacral therapy has been around a long time in both the chiropractic and osteopathic professions, although not all chiropractors and even fewer osteopaths practice it. Many chiropractors use, among other methods, an adjusting technique called *sacral occipital technique.* Within the osteopathic profession there has been a resurgence of interest in craniosacral therapy largely in response to the efforts of Dr. John E. Upledger. The Upledger Institute teaches a comprehensive series of craniosacral classes and while I am not sure how many osteopaths are learning this technique, I can guarantee that legions of physical and massage therapists are.

The cranial bones can become misaligned in a variety of ways, including the very process of being born. In the days before natural birth became popular, many doctors refused to believe that a baby could navigate its way through the birth canal without the help of forceps. Needless to say, grabbing the soft skull of an infant with a large pair of pliers and pulling on it is an excellent way to bestow a cranial misalignment. Even today, while forceps are used much less frequently, there is still the cranial suction cap that pulls on the infant's skull.

Should you manage to survive your birth with your cranial alignment intact, there are always the misadventures of childhood, injuries and accidents that can cause cranial problems. Anyone who has witnessed an infant trying to learn to walk can easily understand how the cranium can become misaligned as the struggling infant spends more time falling down than standing up. During childhood there are a host of possible head injuries that can occur, ranging from innocent falls and sports injuries to, sadly, outright child abuse.

If the craniosacral function is imbalanced, it will translate to spinal imbalance. The cervical spine (aka the neck) that the skull is sitting on and the lower-back/sacral area will be directly affected, and as the mid-back tries to compensate for the imbalances occurring above and below, it too will have trouble staying properly aligned. It is usually quite easy for me to tell whether new patients have a craniosacral problem because they have nearly every box checked off on my form asking about their symptoms.

This brings us back again to that elusive concept of stability, because if the craniosacral function is compromised, patients will not be able to stay in alignment no matter how many times they are treated by their chiropractor. If it turns out that your chiropractor isn't skilled in craniosacral therapy, then you simply need to find a physical or massage therapist who is, and let him or her resolve the imbalance in conjunction with having the chiropractor work on the spinal alignment.

There is no doubt that craniosacral therapy is gaining acceptance within the medical community, as they are referring their patients with neck and back problems to physical therapists who are trained in it. However, if a patient is receiving craniosacral therapy but other parts of the spine are out of alignment, the patient is still going to have to see a chiropractor to gain stability because physical therapists are neither trained nor licensed to perform this manipulation.

From a chiropractic perspective, if your alignment has been correctly evaluated and treated; the Psoas muscle and craniosacral components have been addressed; and you have been given the proper home-care instructions regarding cold compresses, posture, corrective exercises, and stretches; then the *structural component* of your pain syndrome should be well on the road to recovery. The chemical and emotional parts of the health triangle may still need to be considered, but they will be covered in the following chapters.

Unfortunately, in the real world, it doesn't always work that way. As I have stated previously, not every physical disorder is going to respond to chiropractic care, which is why God created orthopedic specialists, acupuncturists, physical therapists, and neurosurgeons. Unless your pain obviously requires surgery, trying chiropractic care first is a safe and conservative approach to getting well. However, there are times when it just doesn't get the job done, and what I try to impress upon my patients is that I don't care *how* they get well, just that they *do* get well. If I can't make it happen through chiropractic, then it is my responsibility to review other options with them.

Acupuncture

As everyone knows, acupuncture has been around for thousands of years and has been used successfully to treat all kinds of ailments in Asian societies. This is another mode of therapy that practitioners of Western medicine don't like because they can't figure out how it works and they aren't trained to perform it. As a result, they disclaim its effectiveness in treating a wide variety of illnesses based on the ever-popular mantra of "where's the research that supports it?"

While much about how acupuncture affects the way the body functions may not be understood, when it comes to suppressing pain, in this area the research is compelling. Acupuncture has the ability to stimulate the release of opiatelike compounds in the brain, thereby blocking the perception of pain. While some Western practitioners want to insist that this is a placebo effect, the fact that Chinese veterinarians use acupuncture as an anesthesia when performing surgery on animals disproves it. Furthermore, when synthetic drugs that block the effects of opiates on brain cells are administered, the effects of acupuncture in relieving pain are lost. So if your pain syndrome is not responding well to chiropractic care, acupuncture can be an excellent option. This is not to say that the two are not compatible; in fact, for very chronic, stubborn problems pursuing acupuncture and chiropractic at the same time can be very beneficial.

Physical Therapy

Another very good approach to relieving pain syndromes may be physical therapy. Sometimes pain is so chronic that patients simply become deconditioned, which is a polite way of saying they get out of shape. If you have been in pain for a long time, it's likely that you have not been able to exercise and the progressive muscle weakness that has ensued may be putting too much stress on your ligaments and joints.

It is also possible that you are suffering from a muscle imbalance, whereby muscles that are supposed to complement and counterbalance each other can't because one has either become too weak or too strong relative to the other one. An example of this problem, which doesn't even involve an injury or pain syndrome, is that of bodybuilders who lift weights unevenly. Without proper training and guidance, some bodybuilders seek to bulk up their "front" muscles. They want strong biceps in their arms and pectorals in their chests, but they neglect to strengthen the opposing muscles because they are less visible (at least to them). This is called *front-loading,* and it leads to joint dysfunction because of the unevenness in strength and disproportionate pulling on the joints.

Physical therapy is also essential in providing rehabilitation of a joint following surgery, such as knee or hip replacement, to make sure the strength and full range of motion is returned to normal.

Physical therapy can also address problems associated with scar tissue. When any connective tissue in the body has been damaged, it will be repaired with scar tissue, whether it is a ligament, tendon, muscle, or your skin. The problem with scar tissue is that it is tougher and less flexible than the original tissue it is repairing and it has more pain-transmitting fibers. At first the tougher-tissue repair sounds like a good idea, but it is not.

Let's say you have a joint whose normal range of motion is ninety degrees, but because of either a serious injury or a series of repetitive injuries, there is a fair amount of what is called *scar-tissue infiltration.* So now you want to move this joint ninety degrees, but the tougher scar tissue embeded along with the normal tissue will only stretch to sixty-five degrees. Then, when you move the joint past sixty-five degrees, the scar tissue tears away from the normal tissue, and because scar tissue has more pain fibers, this is really going to hurt. Now you have another injury that is going to repair with even more scar tissue and probably with more restrictions of motion.

Physical therapy can help scar tissue with a technique known as *remodeling*, which involves breaking up old deposits of scar tissue that have formed in patterns that are not consistent with the direction in which the normal tissue fibers are aligned. With the remodeling process, the old scar tissue is broken down, and the new tissue is modeled to go in the same direction as the normal fibers, thereby increasing flexibility and limiting the chance of further tearing.

ORTHOPEDIC SURGERY

Sometimes physical therapy isn't going to work, and you really need to see an orthopedic surgeon. Some injuries immediately require surgery because the damage is so significant, there is no other option. On the other hand, the problem may be so chronic and advanced that calcium deposits, bone spurs, torn tendons or ligaments, or cartilage degeneration make any kind of recovery impossible without surgical intervention. That doesn't mean that any of the therapies previously described won't have a place in a surgery patient's future, but before any of them can be effective, the damage is going to have to be resolved.

While it is unfortunate that some people truly have suffered permanent physical damage to some parts of their bodies, this is not the case for most of us. Of the people who were in the Merck poll that was discussed at the beginning of this chapter, it is unlikely that many of them were permanently damaged. This means that there is a great deal of hope that the rest of us really can resolve our pain and learn how to keep our bodies healthy.

Actually *resolving* pain syndromes requires more effort and commitment than just reaching for another bottle of pills, but just masking symptoms has far-reaching health consequences that must be considered. It's not only about how you feel today, but about how you will age and what you will have to look forward to as you age. So if you are experiencing pain of any kind, I implore you to try any or all of the therapies I have discussed and don't give up. If you persist, you will most likely make that pain go away, not by masking symptoms, but by treating the cause.

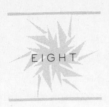

EIGHT

THE NOT-SO-COMMON COMMONSENSE DIET

You're Actually Going to Put *That* in Your Mouth?

ollowing the paradigm of human health consisting of structural, chemical, and mental/emotional integrity, it is time to explore the chemical component. This whole topic can be simplified by breaking it down into which things we put into our bodies that help us and which things that hurt us.

It has been said that nothing is so uncommon as common sense, and I can think of nothing more appropriate than this statement when considering all of the controversy concerning what constitutes a proper diet. The American obsession regarding diet would be hysterically funny were it not for the tragedy of so many people hurting themselves by chasing one crazy diet plan after another. The laughter really stops when we truly comprehend how seriously we are damaging ourselves by the food choices we make on a daily basis.

In Search of the Magic Diet

By virtue of weight-loss programs, diet gurus, and diet-of-the-week fads, the diet business has become a billion-dollar industry as people continually search for the magic diet. We've got protein diets, low-carbohydrate diets, grapefruit diets, diets based on your blood type, rotation diets, liquid diets—basically just about everything except common sense and personal-responsibility diets.

Let me just state that if you are overweight it is because you have an unhealthy emotional relationship with food, a hormonal imbalance, or a combination of the two. Keep in mind that in the human body, one problem can create another problem, which in turn exacerbates the original problem. This is often the case with diet and hormones.

First and foremost, we have to stop pretending that there is some magical diet plan that requires no responsibility on our part and that will make us as slim as some genetically blessed model. We also have to stop thinking that the subject of diet is as complicated as rocket science, because it isn't. What a reasonable diet is is painfully obvious, but for a variety of reasons most people rebel and eat all kinds of garbage.

Without launching into a sociological essay on human behavior, I think the three primary reasons why people eat such an array of unhealthy foods and have such unbalanced diets are: (1) they are conditioned to have an emotional attachment to certain foods; (2) they are bombarded by the relentless advertising and marketing campaigns of the manufacturers of these *food* (and I use the term loosely) products; and (3) they have hormonal imbalances. Unfortunately, all three factors are usually interrelated and perpetrate an unhealthy cycle.

Why a Good Diet Isn't Rocket Science

Let's see just how complex and difficult it is to have a good diet. The human body requires good-quality proteins, carbohydrates, and essential fatty acids to function properly. Since eating is nothing more or less than a refueling of nutrients on a regular basis, it's logical that we should eat good-quality proteins, carbohydrates, and fats in reasonable quantities at each and every meal.

Where in the world we ever got the idea that each meal should be different in its nutritional content is beyond understanding, but in the case of breakfast, I have a strong suspicion that the cereal and bread manufacturers had a lot to do with it.

When you wake up in the morning, your blood sugar is going to be low because you probably haven't eaten anything for nine to twelve hours. It makes absolutely no sense to load your body up with nothing more substantial than a bunch of carbohydrates like cereal, toast, bagels, pastries, or waffles, and then wash it down with juice and caffeinated beverages. These are all foods that will rapidly convert into sugar and precipitate an insulin reaction that will cause you to have low blood sugar a couple of hours later. No wonder you are tired by ten o'clock in the morning and are looking for more sugar and caffeine to give you a jolt! You have also given yourself a great big dose of omega-6 fats, which cause systemic inflammation and cell-wall receptor-site dysfunction (described in Chapter 3).

For blood-sugar stability, a good diet is no more complex than building a fire. To start a fire you need some paper and kindling (carbohydrates) because you need a fast-burning fuel to get things going. However, if at some point you don't start adding logs (protein) for a longer-lasting source of fuel, then either the fire is going to burn out or you will have to keep adding kindling frequently.

This is exactly what happens at breakfast for most people. They eat all kinds of carbohydrate foods that burn up quickly, leaving them tired, irritable, and craving more sugar. Or, even worse, if you plan your life so poorly that you don't have time for breakfast at all, which means you won't be breaking your fast until sometime around lunch-time, you are basically running on empty until noon.

If you have children and are giving them juice, cereal, and a banana to start their day, is it any wonder they might have difficulty staying alert in class or have a tendency to become disruptive? Keep in mind that fruit juices are merely very concentrated amounts of sugar, and be aware that many fruit "juice" products can contain as little as 10 percent real juice while the rest of it is corn syrup and other additives. Even if it is real fruit juice, it might be natural sugar but sugar nonetheless. While most fruits can be very beneficial as a source of fiber, minerals, and vitamins, once you squeeze them into juice, you have lost the fiber and dramatically increased the sugar. When you consider how many oranges you can eat compared to how many you can drink, my point becomes obvious.

If your children begin their day with a carbohydrate high, their blood sugar will begin its rapid descent. To add to the problem, it's pizza and a soda for lunch, with maybe a cookie, and there they go again. By the time these kids see something that resembles protein, it's dinnertime, and by then their blood sugar has been imbalanced throughout most of the day.

THE EMOTIONAL/HORMONAL RELATIONSHIP WITH FOOD

Let's explore the emotional/hormonal relationship with food and how emotions and hormones can work against each other and cause a lot of trouble. When you were a little kid, what were you given if you behaved or did something well? What did your grandparents like to give you just because you were such a little darling? What was always present at holidays such as Halloween, Thanksgiving, Christmas, Easter, Valentine's Day, and birthdays? *Sugar, and lots of it!!* Cakes, candy bars, chocolate bunnies, corn candy, heart-shaped candy, marshmallow chickens, pies—you name it.

It is not hard to imagine how we learned to associate sugar with fun, parties, affection, and reward. We became conditioned to love sugar because it represents positive emotions; it tastes good; and it gives us a short-term glucose high. Looked at in a certain context, it is our first experience with mind-altering substances, and when eaten without enough protein to stabilize blood-sugar levels, it becomes addictive. If this isn't bad enough, many baked goods and processed foods are made with hydrolyzed proteins that contain glutamate, aspartate, and cysteine, chemicals that have an excitatory effect on the brain that makes them as addictive as sugar.

The more sugar you consume, the more insulin your pancreas secretes. Insulin is responsible for enabling sugar to enter the liver, where it will be enzymatically converted into usable glucose or stored as glycogen. It takes time for the liver to make this conversion; in the meantime the blood-sugar level in the body will be low because the insulin has pulled the sugar into the liver. Since the brain's primary fuel is sugar (glucose), it will demand that you eat more sugar when normal levels drop. So you eat more sugar and restart the cycle over and over again.

Perhaps when you were a little kid and your metabolism was more forgiving, or hopefully because you were running around and being physically active, you managed to stay in decent shape. Once you became an adult, a funny thing happened. You slowly but surely realized that you were gaining weight. Somehow that size-six dress is now a size twelve, or the boxer shorts you wore in high school have become large enough to . . . Well, you get the point. What happened?

What happened is that you unwittingly followed the exact program that ranchers use to fatten up farm animals: increased carbohydrate consumption. When you consume more carbohydrates than your body can use, your body *must* store it as fat. The excess carbohydrates cannot be excreted or eliminated through the urine, bowels, or in any other way. The wisdom of this is that carbohydrates stored as fat can be reconverted to glucose in times of famine or extreme physical exertion.

Conversely, if you begin to exercise seriously and restrict your carbohydrate intake, the muscles that are being used will run out of glucose, forcing your body to convert the fat cells back into usable glucose. This is why a good exercise program is essential to weight loss. Unfortunately, if your cortisol levels are imbalanced, you still might not lose weight through exercising because cortisol can cause you to crave and eat more sugar, and it can slow down your ability to burn calories by slowing down your thyroid-gland function.

Because appropriately restricting certain carbohydrates should help you lose weight, there are now diets that propose the elimination of *all* carbohydrates. The idea is to eat all the bacon, eggs, cheese, and steak you want. What could be more fun than that? Heck, you didn't like all of those vegetables your parents tried to make you eat when you were a kid anyway. In all fairness, most diets that advocate a high quantity of protein do add carbohydrates after two or three weeks, but people often misinterpret the need for carbohydrates and think they will lose more weight if they simply stick with only eating protein.

The problem with eating mostly protein is that it can cause liver and kidney disorders, atherosclerosis (plaque in your arteries), and possibly diabetes. The absence of carbohydrates will mean a severe reduction in insulin, and if this occurs for a lengthy period of time, the liver will form substances called *ketones* and *acetones* that will harm the kidneys and liver. Similarly, a prolonged reduction of insulin can cause an elevation of cholesterol, which can increase the risk of atherosclerosis and heart disease.

So, you are still overweight and in search of the magical diet plan that will return your body to its glorious youth, unless you got a head start and became overweight as a child. You are resisting exercise because it takes up a lot of time and energy, and besides, you mow the lawn once a week and, in your mind, that should count for something. Not only that, but you work really hard, and your boss, spouse, and kids are driving you crazy, and you could use a little reward for being such a good person.

What could be better than an ultrarefined carbohydrate called alcohol to make those stresses go away? Or maybe a handful of M&M's or Hershey's Kisses? Häagen-Dazs anyone? Your daily diet doesn't support your blood sugar right from the start of your day, which makes you too tired to exercise, and you are cranky and so stressed out that your cortisol level is constantly pushing the reward button in your brain that says you not only need that candy bar, but by God you *deserve* it! You have been conditioned to associate sugar with happiness and rewards; you could use a little happiness and reward.

The only problem is that the rewards are making you gain weight day after day, and that by itself is becoming pretty stressful. When you look in the mirror, you are not particularly proud of what you see, and soon you will have to deal with your doctor warning you of the risks of heart problems and/or diabetes With all of this stress, what's a person to do? In all probability, you are going to respond to the need for immediate gratification and have another drink, candy bar, or ice cream cone, and decide that tomorrow will be the great day of change and reformation. Okay, maybe not tomorrow but certainly next week. Oh wait, that won't work because that's when your vacation, birthday, or the holidays are coming up and that wouldn't be a good time to start a diet.

There are four things that have to happen to reverse this unhealthy cycle:

1. Have your cortisol levels checked with an adrenal stress index test and also have your insulin and glucose levels checked.
2. Adopt a common-sense diet guided by knowledge regarding the foods you eat.
3. Make a commitment to regular physical exercise.
4. Arrive at a true understanding of your emotional/psychological relationship with food and decide that you don't want to be a pawn for every clever advertisement that promises you thrills, fun, or sex because you consume their beer, burgers, or soda.

It is very important to reiterate that if your cortisol levels are imbalanced, and especially if the cause is intestinal inflammation, you will not get well, lose weight, or be able to keep your diet under control. If your cortisol levels are imbalanced, you will intellectually know you are doing all of the wrong things, and you will even feel guilty about it, but the cortisol will make you do them anyway. It truly is sad to see some people try so hard and fail, when all that is wrong is their cortisol levels. Please get yours checked before you even bother with anything else, and refer to the previous chapter for ways to resolve these imbalances.

The following dietary recommendations are, of necessity, generalized. This means that this diet concept will work for most people most of the time. Just as I made the point at the beginning of this book that people respond to stress differently, it is difficult to find the one diet plan that will work for every single human being. If you have a specific illness or genetic disorder, then you should already be consulting with a nutritionist familiar with your special needs.

In the beginning of this chapter, I promised you that having a good diet did not have to be rocket science and could be straightforward and easy to understand. I have found in my own practice that many people really do try to follow a good diet plan, but that some diets are so complicated and difficult to comprehend, with odd measurements and point systems, that they just give up and order a pizza with a diet soda.

The goal of any good diet is to have good-quality proteins, carbohydrates, and fats in appropriate amounts and in fixed ratios with each other. Let's take each food group in order and see how easy it is to incorporate them into a healthy, balanced diet.

PROTEINS

The first easy rule regarding proteins is that the National Research Council recommends that you calculate your daily protein requirement in grams by taking your weight and dividing it by two. This means that if you weigh 140 pounds, then you will need 70 grams of protein per day. If you are very physically active you may require a little more, and if you are trying to lose weight by increasing your level of exercise, then you won't.

The second easy rule about proteins and grams is that per ounce, all meat proteins are the same. This means that one ounce of chicken, beef, pork, lamb, or turkey all average 7 grams of protein per ounce.

Conveniently, one egg equals 7 grams of protein. Even fish is pretty close to this average, with a range of 5 to 7 grams of protein per ounce.

So, if you require 70 grams of protein per day, you can have 10 ounces of meat or fish daily, or 8 ounces if you have two eggs for breakfast. Since this is supposed to be a commonsense diet, it presumes you will choose lean cuts of meat that are not loaded with fat and not assume pork means bacon or sausage.

A lot of people get a little testy about how are they are supposed to know how many ounces a piece of meat or fish is without getting their old kitchen scale out. Fortunately, we live in such a great country that it is nearly impossible to buy any protein in a market that does not have the weight listed right on the package.

So let's say you go to the market and buy a package of four skinless chicken breasts for dinner that weigh 1 pound. This would mean that each chicken breast weighs 4 ounces (and contains 28 grams of protein), so you still need six more ounces (or 42 grams) of protein to fulfill your daily requirement (if you require 70 grams of protein).

For lunch you grab a can of tuna, and the label tells you it weighs 6 ounces. If you eat half of the can, you still have three more ounces of protein to go. This means that for breakfast you could have two eggs and get very close to your total protein requirement. In reality, you will probably get there easily because there will be a few grams of protein in the bread you are likely to put the tuna on or in the toast you have with your eggs.

There are also other types of protein that are going to be in your diet, and you need to know how to figure them into how much you may consume. Somehow, with proteins, seven seems to be the lucky number. One cup of milk or yogurt equals 7 grams of protein. A half cup of beans or peas equals 7 grams of protein, as does 1 ounce of almonds or peanuts.

So if you pay just a little attention to the weight of the protein foods you are buying, you should have very little difficulty figuring out how much you should eat. You can also make it less difficult by buying in quantities that are easy to calculate. Instead of buying two-thirds of a pound of lunch meat, buy either a half or a whole pound.

CARBOHYDRATES

Unlike its guidelines for proteins, the National Research Council has no specific daily requirements for how many carbohydrates an individual should consume, and this is the part of the diet that people struggle with most, both in terms of which kinds and how many carbohydrates they should be eating.

In order to make intelligent choices about which carbohydrates you should eat, you need to be aware that not all carbohydrates are absorbed the same way. Some are more quickly digested and the resulting sugars released more rapidly into the bloodstream. A particular carbohydrate's ability to raise blood-sugar levels is assigned a numerical value called the *glycemic index*. The carbohydrates that have the highest numerical value are the ones that will cause the greatest output of insulin and thus lead to weight gain, fatigue, and increased carbohydrate cravings. Carbohydrates that enter the bloodstream very quickly and raise blood-sugar levels abruptly will cause an elevated insulin response, which in turn will actually result in low blood sugar as the excess insulin performs its task of whisking the sugar off to the liver to be processed into glucose. At this point, the low blood sugar will make you crave more sugar, and you restart the negative cycle all over again. Keep in mind that any sugar your body doesn't burn up with activity gets stored away as fat for future use.

Now I could torture you with an extensive list of the glycemic index of every carbohydrate, but that simply isn't necessary. It will be a lot easier if we just think in terms of "helpful" carbohydrates and "unhelpful" ones. The "unhelpful" carbohydrates are bread, pasta, grains, potatoes, carrots, corn, cereals, rice and rice cakes, papayas, bananas, raisins and other dried fruits, and most fruit juices. Does this mean you are never going to eat them again? Of course not, but it does mean that you should eat them less frequently and in smaller amounts.

The "helpful" carbohydrates are obviously everything else that's left, but even then, some are better than others. In the following lists we will divide the rest of the carbohydrates into two groups: The first group contains the ones that will affect your blood-sugar levels the least, and those will be the carbohydrates that you want to eat the most; the second group contains the carbohydrates you may still eat, but in moderation.

Best Carbohydrates

Broccoli	Celery	Yellow squash
Spinach	Lettuce	Black beans
Cabbage	(not iceberg)	Okra
Peppers	Turnip	Cherries
Mushrooms	Eggplant	Grapefruit
Zucchini	Tomato	Apricots
Green beans	Cauliflower	Orange
Onions	Endive	Kiwi
Lentils	Kidney beans	Blueberries
Asparagus	Collard greens	Tangerine
Bok choy	Swiss chard	Peach
Kale	Cucumber	Nectarine
Brussels sprouts	Bean sprouts	Pear
Leeks	Radishes	Pineapple
Artichoke	Sauerkraut	Apple

Second-Best Carbohydrates

Beets	Parsnip
Lima beans	Peas
Acorn squash	Sweet potato
Butternut squash	

Perhaps you have noticed the glaring absence of certain carbohydrates, such as carrots, corn, potatoes, rice, and pasta. The reason for this is that in an ideal diet, you want to avoid these carbohydrates, because they are all very high on the glycemic index, and in the case of corn, potatoes, and pasta, they can increase systemic inflammation. Does this mean you will never eat corn on the cob or a baked potato again? Of course not, but it does mean you should have them infrequently and not make them staples of your diet.

Now that we have established a hierarchy of carbohydrates, we need to determine how much you can eat to maintain a balance with your protein consumption. If you are eating from the Best Carbohydrate list, then a good rule of thumb is to have twice as much carbohydrate as protein. You can usually do this with a simple visual assessment. When you also consider that all of the "helpful" carbohydrates are loaded with fiber, vitamins, and minerals, it really is hard to eat too much to the point where it would be detrimental to your health.

When determining the amount of second-best or "unhelpful" carbohydrates to consume, you want to keep the ratios even, so that the amount of carbohydrate appears to be about the same as the amount of protein. For example, if you are having half of a chicken breast, then half of a baked potato would look about right. A mound of rice or pasta that is the same size as the protein serving would be okay.

You also want to make sure that you don't have two "unhelpful" carbohydrates in the same meal. You don't want to combine corn, carrots, beets, potatoes, rice, or pasta because they will overload the glycemic index of the meal. A classic example of this is Thanksgiving dinner, when sweet potatoes, bread stuffing, mashed potatoes, glazed carrots, and pumpkin pie conspire to a crescendo of blood-sugar disaster and leave the participants lying semiconscious on the sofa. So the best choice you can make when putting a meal together is to have a reasonable amount of lean protein with good, fresh vegetables or fruits from the "helpful" carbohydrate list.

The stickler in this program for most people has to do with bread and what to eat for breakfast. It isn't too difficult to figure out what to eat for dinner if you are choosing the correct amounts of chicken, fish, beef, pork, or tofu with "helpful" carbohydrates. Even lunch isn't too challenging if you choose a sandwich of whole-grain bread with a good amount of protein and lettuce and tomato, a hearty soup, or a salad with protein in it. But we have become so conditioned to a carbohydrate-laden breakfast that it is difficult to figure out what type of protein sounds appealing first thing in the morning.

One obvious choice would be eggs, but you can't eat them seven days a week, and there is the time problem of having to cook them. Other good choices include low-fat cottage cheese or low-fat yogurt with fruit. (With yogurt it is important to read the label and see how much sugar is in it.) Ideally, you want to stay with plain yogurt and add your own fruit because the fruit preserves in yogurt are loaded with sugar. A slice of whole-grain bread with natural peanut butter (make sure it is not the typical grocery-store variety with hydrogenated oils and sugar added to it) or almond butter is another option.

My favorite recommendation to the time-challenged, don't-know-what-to-eat-for-breakfast person is a protein drink. Protein powders can be bought in any health food store (many grocery stores also sell them), and they can be made from egg whites, whey, or soy. They can be strictly protein or they can also contain carbohydrates, which basically makes them a complete meal. How you decide which one to purchase depends on what you plan to mix it with. If you are going to mix the powder with water or milk, you will want the kind with carbohydrates added in order to keep your nutrients balanced. If you are going to add fruit or fruit juice to it, then you might want to stick to the protein-only powder. My advice is to use a blender and make a quart at a time to store in the refrigerator. That way you won't be washing the blender every day, and it will be conveniently waiting for you in the morning. Just drink it and go, no muss and no fuss.

FATS

This is the really easy part once you put the onion dip away. Your body does need essential fatty acids to function normally, and the best way to get these is from fish. Other than that, you should use only olive oil, unless you absolutely have to deep-fry something, and then I would recommend soybean or peanut oil. You do not want to use canola or vegetable oils, and you do want to learn how to make your own salad dressing and avoid the store-bought varieties. If you cannot find the time to whisk together some olive oil, vinegar, and herbs, then you need to reassess your life.

The topic of omega-6 versus omega-3 fats has recently become enormously important in medical research because of the far-reaching health problems related to excessive dietary omega-6 fats. If you re-call from Chapter 3, omega-6 oils cause inflammation by converting arachidonic acid into prostaglandin-E2, which is a highly inflamma-tory chemical. The omega-6 fats, which come from corn oil, hydro-genated oils, meat, most baked goods, margarine, and deep-fried foods, have been scientifically linked to coronary heart disease and el-evated cholesterol, atherosclerosis, thrombosis, systemic inflammation, Alzheimer's disease, rheumatoid arthritis and other autoimmune dis-orders, and receptor-site dysfunction that inhibits neurotransmitter attachment to the cell membrane and in so doing can result in psy-chiatric disorders and hormonal imbalances. Given the fact that the American diet is *loaded* with omega-6 oils (on any given day in the United States about one-quarter of the adult population visits a fast-food restaurant, and Americans spend more than $110 billion a year on fast food, which is more than they spend on movies, books, mag-azines, newspapers, videos, and recorded music combined), is it any wonder we are one of the sickest nations on the planet?

Because of my obvious concern regarding inflammation and its ef-fect on human health, I find the current interest and research fasci-nating, but I also see an inevitable and ugly showdown looming in the future. It's like two huge trains on the same track heading toward each other: One train is bona fide medical research, and the other is the fast-food industry, which includes the soft-drink industry. This pits research that says this junk food is making us sick and even psychiat-rically disturbed against McDonalds, Burger King, Coca-Cola, Pepsi, etc. Coca-Cola has launched a multimillion-dollar campaign in which Tom Cruise directed Penelope Cruz in a commercial to portray the drink as "natural and relevant." This is a product that is loaded with corn (omega-6) sugar because it's cheaper than cane sugar, and caffeine, and has no nutritional benefit whatsoever. How is that "natural and relevant"? It will be fascinating to watch how the fast-food as well as the processed-food industries will try to advertise themselves out of this controversy.

Beyond the obvious need to avoid foods that are high in omega-6 oils, the cure to all of this lies in consuming omega-3 oils, which are in pumpkin seeds, walnuts, beans, soy products, and most significantly, fish and fish oils. Most research indicates that omega-3 from fish oil is easily assimilated in the body. Omega-3 oils protect the vascular system, reduce inflammation in the brain, have a specific role in brain development and regeneration of nerve cells, reduce the risk of coronary heart disease and cardiac arrhythmia, relieve the pain and swelling in rheumatoid arthritis, and inhibit autoimmune reactions.

While there is no known RDA (recommended daily allowance) for omega-3 oils, research studies on rheumatoid arthritis used doses of 1,500 mg with good results. If you have a good diet, a daily dose of 1,000 mg per day seems like a reasonable amount. If your diet isn't too wonderful just yet, or you are at risk of heart disease or depression, you might want to go as high as 4,000 mg per day. Recent research indicates that an increase in omega-3 oils might result in a depletion of antioxidants in the body, so it is important to take antioxidant vitamins when taking omega-3 oils. Antioxidants are so essential to human health, you should be taking them anyway. The antioxidant vitamins are E, A, C, and grape seed extract, and I'll go into further detail on this subject in this chapter.

Other good sources of fat are avocados, tahini (sesame seed butter), and raw nuts. When necessary, you should always use butter instead of margarine, since one is actually a food and the other is not. Which brings us to our next category.

Things You Shouldn't Put in Your Mouth

Remarkably, human beings eat all kinds of garbage that can't even be classified as food, and about 90 percent of the money Americans spend on food is used to buy processed food. What exactly is the nutritional value of coffee or soda? Zero would be the correct answer. And what of "foods" that have been so overprocessed as to be devoid of any nutritional benefit, such as potato chips, cheese puffs, fast foods, and lots of wonderful convenience foods found in your supermarket's freezer whose ingredients would require that you have a degree in chemistry to figure out what they actually are? Beyond the problem of the omega-6 oils previously discussed, there are the problems of free radicals and excitotoxins in processed foods. Excitotoxins are glutamate (not to be confused with glutamine), aspartate, and cysteine, which are commonly used as flavor enhancers (e.g., monosodium glutamate or MSG) and artificial sweeteners. Excitotoxins are frequently diguised by labeling them as "hydrolyzed protein," and you should avoid consuming these products.

The human body is a dynamic masterpiece of chemical interactions, and how we have come to a place where we routinely put all manner of toxic trash into our bodies is completely beyond comprehension. Earlier in this chapter I noted the many different types of diets that are based on so many conflicting rationales. Most of these diets do have one thing in common as far as weight loss is concerned, and that is that they work, as long as the dieter doesn't have hormonal imbalances. The reason for this is that they all share a common thread, which is the avoidance of processed and refined foods. It's as simple as that!

Whether it's the Atkins low-carbohydrate/high-protein diet, or the Zone 40-30-30 (ratio of carbohydrates to protein to fats) diet, or the *Eat Right for Your Type* (a different diet for different blood types) diet, or the McDougall high-carbohydrate/low-protein diet, they all forbid junk food. All of these diets eliminate refined flours, refined sugars, hydrogenated oils, and food additives and preservatives. By doing away with all of this garbage and eating real food in reasonable amounts, people are bound to lose weight.

Now that you know which foods can help you and which ones can sabotage your efforts to have a diet that is nutritionally and hormonally supportive, next comes the commonsense part.

FOOD AS FUEL

The concept that you really have to embrace is that eating represents a fuel-delivery system to your body. It's not enough to stuff any old thing into your stomach to relieve the sensation of hunger; the goal is to provide your body with the correct balance of nutrients that will keep you healthy and vital every single day. Unfortunately, most people don't approach their diets this way, even though they intellectually know better.

For a useful analogy, compare your need for fuel to that of your car. When your body is getting low on fuel your brain creates the sensation of hunger, which triggers the desire for food. With regard to your stomach, you are trying to go from empty to full. Your car's fuel gauge does the same thing, but instead of the physical sensations that let you know when it's time to refuel, there is an indicator to make you aware of the level of gas in the tank.

So let's say that one day it's time to rush off to work and, oops, your car's fuel gauge indicates that it is very close to empty and you will run out of gas before you get to work. You are going to have to take some action to bring the gauge from empty to full. Well, maybe you don't really have the time to drive to the gas station, so why not grab the garden hose and fill the tank with water? Or you could run back into the house and get a couple of half gallons of soda and pour them into the tank. Either way you are adding fluid to a gauge that measures liquid content, and if you turn the ignition key to just the place where the electrical system engages, you are going to see the needle go from E (empty) to F (full). Mission accomplished! What's that you say? This is the stupidest thing you have ever heard of because putting any old liquid into the fuel tank will destroy the engine and render the car useless.

This is no different from dumping some sugar-coated product and a cup of caffeine into your stomach to create the sensation of "full" and thinking that you're going to end up in any better condition than your car will. The only difference is that your car will die immediately, whereas your body will let you get away with this foolishness for a while. And whereas you can always buy another car, it is not likely that science will advance to the point that you can buy another body in the near future.

The commonsense approach to a healthy diet is to ask yourself "Is this going to be good for me or bad for me?" Is the next thing you put in your mouth going to represent usable fuel or just a bunch of toxins your liver is going to have to figure out how to get rid of? Does putting a particular substance into your stomach make any sense, or is it just as stupid as putting water or soda into your car's gas tank?

As straightforward and simplistic as all this may sound, at the heart of the problem are the intangible quirks of human nature: It is usually easier to lie to ourselves that one more day of a bad diet won't matter, and immediate gratification supersedes long-range common sense.

As a daily reminder of why a healthy diet is a good idea, you could vividly imagine what you will look and feel like if you keep eating garbage day after day, year after year into the future. To this end, start noticing the elderly people you encounter in the grocery store, the mall, or the bank. Some of them will be fit and vital, physically capable of leading active lives, while others will be so overweight and in such poor condition that they use the grocery cart as a walker.

While I realize that in the above example there are multiple factors in addition to diet that influence how we will age, such as genetics, injury, and diseases, diet is the one factor we have control of most of the time. There are instances, however, when we're not in control.

Hormone Imbalances Cause Food Cravings

I know I sounded harsh with this commonsense and personal-responsibility perspective, so it's time for a little sympathy. The dynamics of how people gain weight remain consistent, but what initiates the dynamics varies. For some it can be that they have developed an unhealthy psychological relationship to food and they are using it as a crutch, while for others it can be that they just got unlucky with an injury or a disease that caused them to take long-term NSAIDs or antibiotics, which resulted in the leaky-gut/high-cortisol syndrome and blood-sugar imbalances. In either case, whether the stress hormones are psychologically or physiologically induced, the food cravings that result are very real.

As I have already mentioned, stress hormones dominate the neurotransmitters of rational thought. So even though you logically know that candy bar is not going to make you feel or look any better, if your hormones are imbalanced, you will be driven to eat it. This is what happens to people who attempt to faithfully follow diet programs but find themselves cheating or, worse, find that they don't lose much weight because their hormonal metabolic rate will not cooperate. By following the program discussed in Chapter 6 on how to correct hormone imbalances, you will be able to regain hormone stability so that you can be in control of what you choose to eat.

Another point that I want to make is that we are not expecting to achieve sainthood with regard to our diet; we are seeking balance and good health. Does this mean you will never have an ice cream cone, a martini, or a bonbon again? Of course not! What it means is that you will consume food responsibly with a conscious awareness of the nutrients you are fueling your body with most of the time. If your diet is good 85 percent of the time, you can certainly allow yourself to indulge in the occasional treat. The problem is when over half of the stuff you consume hardly even qualifies as nutritious food (such as meals from fast-food restaurants), or when the food choices you make are so imbalanced they compromise your internal chemistry.

THE PRO-INFLAMMATORY STATE AND DIETARY FACTORS OF PAIN

There are three reasons why a good diet is pertinent to this discussion of cortisol imbalances. A poor diet can cause: (1) spinal and peripheral joint pain; (2) hormonal imbalances; and (3) leaky-gut syndrome. As we have seen in the previous chapters, these three problems can be intimately related and perpetuate each other.

There is not a chiropractor or medical doctor in the world who has not encountered patients in severe pain who insist that there was no physical activity on their part that would cause that level of suffering. They didn't lift anything; they weren't gardening or washing the car; they weren't even bending over and reaching for something. Their stress levels are fine, and they weren't even thinking evil thoughts. Suddenly, out of the blue, their back went into spasm and now they can barely move.

This is the time for the doctor to ask the patient what he or she has been eating, because dietary imbalances can cause the body to go into the pro-inflammatory state of systemic inflammation, which can cause irritation of the pain neurons inside the joints. The pro-inflammatory state describes an increase in substances that exist naturally in the body but become chemical irritants at excessively high levels. The substances that cause the most problems are: lactic acid, histamine, prostaglandin-E2, bradykinin, and arachidonic acid.

A diet that is deficient in certain vitamins or minerals can result in an excess of these chemical irritants. Similarly, a diet that is too high in fats, caffeine, and toxins will also cause an increase in the pro-inflammatory chemicals. The pro-inflammatory state is characterized by increased tissue acidity; increased free radicals, which means unstable molecules; fatty-acid imbalance; and insufficient mineral intake, particularly potassium.

What happens is that a poor diet elevates levels of these substances to the point where they irritate the pain nerve fibers inside of the joints, which in turn will trigger intense muscle spasms. The muscle spasms then further distort the alignment of the joint, meaning that they restrict the ability of the joint to move in its normal manner, which further irritates the nerves in the joint. It's another one of those circular problems when things go from bad to worse.

A good example, something that I see several times a year in my practice, involves arachidonic acid. Foods that contain arachidonic acid are beef, pork, lamb, dairy, shrimp, lobster, clams, and, worst of all, hydrogenated oils/trans-fats. I live and practice on the California coast, where there is a propensity toward seafood consumption. So every now and then when I get patients who have intense back pain and can't think of a single reason for it, I amaze them with my psychic skills by asking them if they have been eating a lot of shellfish lately. They look at me with astonishment and then go on to tell me that their market was having a great sale on shrimp or prawns and that they have been eating them for days.

The Importance of a Balanced pH

Let's look at each factor of the pro-inflammatory state with regard to what causes it and how to correct it. First, we have increased tissue acidity, which, as a consequence of improper eating habits, disables the body's buffer systems from maintaining a normal acid–alkaline balance. This balance of acid/alkaline content in the blood and tissues is referred to as the body's *pH*. It has been established that people with a proper tissue pH will heal more rapidly from an injury than those without a proper pH. The normal range of intracellular pH is 6.0 to 7.4, and an elevation beyond that range is called *acidosis*.

While the body's pH is generally kept in check by the lungs and the kidneys, the foods you consume on a daily basis do have a great influence on the acid/alkaline balance. The acid-forming foods are meat, dairy, fish, and grains. The alkaline-forming foods are fruits and

vegetables in general, which means that there are some fruits and vegetables that can be a little acidic.

Once again we come to that horribly boring concept of balance
as the key to good health, but it is easy to see how a diet that has a
good balance of proteins, carbohydrates, and fats will also keep the
pH within normal range. By not consuming to many acid-forming
foods, you will keep the levels of lactic acid and bradykinins within a
normal, noninflammatory range.

Bradykinin is a potent chemical irritant, whose importance in
joint pain was demonstrated in 1967, when a researcher named Mel-
mon discovered its presence in the fluid of arthritic joints. Bradykinin
exists throughout the body, including the joints and surrounding soft
tissue, and is elevated either by injury or by diet. So while a diet that
promotes tissue acidity and elevations of bradykinin can initiate pain,
the situation can be made even worse by suffering a physical injury
and then compromising the recovery with an acidic diet.

Free Radicals

The next factor in the pro-inflammatory state is free radicals, which
consist of an atom or group of atoms with an unpaired electron. Free
radicals work like a game of musical chairs, when the last person left
standing when the music stops is the loser. In the game of free-radical
musical chairs, the atom that is left unpaired attempts to disturb the
molecular balance of the other atoms.

Free radicals damage protein molecules, DNA, and the protective
lipid (fat) barrier that surrounds each cell. They have been linked to
many diseases, including cancer, but they are also a normal by-product
of digestion. The body's ability to rid itself of free radicals depends on
another group of chemicals called *antioxidants,* but problems can occur if there are too many free radicals. In a research article titled "The
Support for a Role for Antioxidants in Reducing Cancer," the author,
G. Block, states: "Without continuous and abundant antioxidant and
radical scavenging capability, survival would be impossible."

From the perspective of diet, the greatest risk of elevated free radicals comes from eating processed foods that contain all kinds of chemicals that have nothing to do with nutrition. These chemicals are used for the manufacturer's benefit to hold the product together; enhance its shelf life; or affect its color, texture, or taste. In your body they are toxins that your liver is going to have to work hard to get rid of. The danger is that these free radicals can disrupt the normal molecular arrangement of your cells and cause them to malfunction. In terms of pain, free radicals irritate joints and soft tissues such as muscles and ligaments.

Fatty Acid Imbalance

The role of omega-6 oils in causing inflammation has already been discussed, so I am just going to briefly remind you that the main problem with them is that they convert arachidonic acid into prostaglandin-E2, which is a highly inflammatory chemical that irritates the body's tissues.

One example of why essential fatty acids, such as omega-6 and omega-3 oils, figure in the pro-inflammatory state and the production of pain involves the body's ability to heal and repair itself on a continuous basis. The role of fatty acids in repairing damaged intervertebral discs in the spine is discussed in a research article titled "Nutrition and the Biochemistry of the Intervertebral Disc" by J. Siekerka. The article states: "Nutritional therapy should accompany any chosen treatment regime to accelerate the disc's healing process. The most integral aspect of acute therapy appears to be the dietary addition of foods high in essential fatty acids and the elimination of foods that contain arachidonic acid." If the protective membranes of your cells cannot effectively repair and maintain their integrity, the tissue will become weakened and more prone to injury. A more recent research study found that elevated levels of prostaglandin-E2 are a major factor in lumbar disc herniations and that a diet low in omega-6 oils and high in omega-3 oils can protect the disc by preventing the conversion of arachidonic acid to prostaglandin-E2.

MINERAL DEFICIENCIES

The last factor in the pro-inflammatory state is mineral deficiency. Because there are so many minerals required to maintain normal body function, we will concentrate only on those whose deficiencies can play a role in pain. The four minerals most likely to be involved in this process are calcium, magnesium, potassium, and zinc.

Calcium

Many people are aware that too little calcium will upset muscle metabolism and bone stability. A while back I stated that, for the most part, muscles only do what the nerves tell them to do and don't just decide to contract on their own. I made this point because a frequent problem in trying to correct a pain syndrome is attempting to treat the muscle instead of the neurological factors (spinal-joint nerve irritation) that cause the muscles to become overly tense or spastic.

The exception in this case is a mineral imbalance, which can cause a muscle spasm, in most cases as a result of insufficient calcium. When a muscle connected to the spine goes into spasm, it will very likely cause spinal-joint nerve irritation, which will prolong the spasm because the nerve supply to the muscle is no longer functioning normally. Dietary calcium can be best acquired by eating green leafy vegetables, dairy products, shellfish, and molasses, and the minimum daily requirement should be 1,000 mg a day.

Magnesium

Magnesium is also essential to muscle function and critically important to normal heart function. Low levels of magnesium have been associated with fibromyalgia, chronic fatigue syndrome, heart disease, and muscle cramps. I know this will come as a big surprise to you, but one of the leading factors in magnesium depletion is stress. This is because the adrenal glands' secretion of aldosterone regulates the rate of magnesium excretion through the kidneys, which is increased by stress.

Magnesium influences how nutrients pass through cell membranes by regulating electrical charges and activating the enzymes required for protein and carbohydrate metabolism. It is also an important factor in regulating the body's acid/alkaline balance. Because the cooking process destroys magnesium, magnesium deficiencies are more common than you might imagine. Other causes of low magnesium levels are antibiotics, alcohol consumption, diuretics, and a high-carbohydrate diet.

This leads us to another bizarre scenario that illustrates how things can go so wrong when viewed from the wrong perspective. Let's say that, for whatever reason, you become seriously stressed-out. By now you know all of the dynamics of what your adrenal glands are going to do, and you know your blood sugar and magnesium levels are going to be lowered. So you start craving sweets, which leads you to the high-carbohydrate diet, and possibly you drink more alcohol to dull the stress. This poor diet, of course, only continues to lower your magnesium levels, which can ultimately precipitate a heart attack (although the adrenal stress could do that all by itself by constricting your coronary blood vessels).

A frequent part of the medical management of heart disease is diuretics, which will lower magnesium levels even more while also lowering your blood pressure. The adrenal-gland function has not been addressed, nor has your diet, nor your alcohol consumption, and now you are taking drugs that will cause you to lose more magnesium, which may set you up for your next heart attack. This state of affairs will mean that you will be prescribed aspirin on a daily basis, which brings us back to intestinal-tract inflammation, elevated cortisol levels, and a continuation of all of your problems with no end in sight. Sometimes the merry-go-round doesn't stop, and you can literally find that your health problems are going around in circles.

The best sources of magnesium are *raw* green leafy vegetables (spinach, arrugula, salad greens), soybeans, seeds and nuts (especially almonds), figs, unmilled wheat germ, and milk. The minimum daily requirement of magnesium is 400 mg per day.

Potassium

Potassium deficiency has been linked to high blood pressure, strokes, diabetes, and muscle pain and weakness. As it relates to the pro-inflammatory state, potassium deficiency can cause an elevation in prostaglandin-E2, which irritates the joints. Because the adrenal mineralocorticoids (aldosterone) are responsible for maintaining and balancing the minerals in the body, potassium can suffer the same fate as magnesium and be lost through the urine in times of stress.

Other causes of potassium deficiencies are excessive salt intake, a diet high in refined sugar, and a diet that is lacking enough fruits and vegetables. Alcohol and caffeine increase the urinary excretion of potassium.

Potassium occurs in many different foods, including meats, vegetables, fruits, sunflower seeds, and beans, so it is not hard to get it through your diet. A minimum of 2,500 mg of potassium should be consumed daily, but the problem with potassium is not so much getting it in your diet as it is keeping it inside your body. Thus, we come back to managing stress effectively and having a good diet that supports hormonal balance.

Zinc

Zinc becomes important in the pro-inflammatory state by virtue of its ability to inhibit the release from the mast cells of histamine, which precipitates the inflammatory process. Anyone who has ever had a cold is familiar with the effects of histamine, the agent that causes all of the swelling and congestion that is part of having a cold. It's a valuable agent because it does help to initiate the immune response that will defend your body from viruses and bacteria, but when histamine is released with tissue injuries, it promotes inflammation that is not desirable.

Zinc deficiency is usually the result of eating processed foods or foods that are grown in zinc-depleted soil. A diet that is high in natural, unprocessed foods is likely to have adequate amounts of zinc in it. Diets that contain good proteins, wheat bran and germ, nuts, spinach, mushrooms, and pumpkin seeds are high in zinc. The minimum daily requirement is 15 mg, and you need to be careful to not overdo it because too much zinc can cause a loss of iron and copper.

In addition to the importance of keeping your body out of the pro-inflammatory state by having a good diet, there are natural supplements you can take to reduce inflammation. This is very important because none of these supplements have the damaging effects on the intestinal tract that NSAIDs do. These supplements are collectively known as *proteolytic enzymes,* and they are exceptionally good at reducing inflammation, relieving pain, and speeding up the healing process.

PROTEOLYTIC ENZYMES

These are enzymes that cause a chemical chain reaction in the body to break down proteins. One of the very best proteolytic enzymes is bromelain, which is a naturally occurring enzyme found in pineapples. Research has shown that bromelain reduces bradykinin production, thus lowering its ability to irritate the pain fibers in joints. The most powerful of the pro-inflammatory irritants, bradykinin, can cause pain and swelling, activate other pain-producing prostaglandins, and promote fibrous scar tissue, so being able to reduce it with bromelain is truly significant.

Other proteolytic enzymes that reduce inflammation and pain are papain and pancreatin. Most vitamin stores sell bromelain either separately or in combination with these other enzymes, and I think that taking them all together will achieve the best results. These proteolytic enzymes *must* be taken on an empty stomach, or they will just assist with the digestion of your food and not reach the sites of inflammation. These supplements have no known negative side effects, so you can take rather large amounts.

Each manufacturer may vary the amount of each proteolytic enzyme contained in each pill, but on average there will be 50 mg of bromelain, 50 mg of papain, and 50 mg of pancreatin. Initially I would recommend five pills five times a day, and after two weeks I would reduce it to three pills three times a day until the condition is resolved.

There are other supplements to consider in treating the pro-inflammatory state such as ginger, turmeric, and antioxidants.

Ginger is a wonderful anti-inflammatory agent because it has the dual properties of reducing the prostaglandins that cause inflammation while at the same time protecting the lining of the stomach. You will recall that the whole problem with NSAIDs is that they irritate the gastrointestinal lining and can cause the leaky-gut/elevated-cortisol syndrome. Ginger can be as effective as NSAIDs in relieving joint swelling and stiffness, but it will not damage the intestinal lining and, in fact, will protect it.

Ginger can be consumed in many ways, ranging from the fresh root used to season foods, to teas, to capsules of dried ginger powder. The capsules are the most potent form of ginger and realistically the easiest way to consistently get it into your system. An effective dosage would be 1,000 mg taken four times a day with food.

Turmeric, also a good anti-inflammatory herb, has been shown in research studies to be as effective as cortisone and ibuprofen. The active ingredient in turmeric is curcumin. Turmeric is widely used in curry dishes and is easy to find in any grocery store as a seasoning. It can also be obtained in capsule form in health food and vitamin stores. An appropriate amount would be 50 mg twice a day with food.

The only drawback to taking turmeric is that it is believed to be effective because it raises the level of cortisol, which accounts for its anti-inflammatory effect. If you only have an acute or recent injury and don't suffer from all of the negative effects of high cortisol levels that I have described thus far (e.g., insomnia, depression, sugar and/ or salt cravings), then it is safe to take for approximately two weeks. If your pain is more chronic or if you have the other symptoms of elevated cortisol, I would recommend that you use the ginger and proteolytic enzymes instead of the turmeric.

ANTIOXIDANTS

Antioxidants remove free radicals from the body, and the most widely known antioxidant is vitamin C, which performs many valuable functions: It is essential in connective-tissue repair; it protects the body against infection; it enhances the level of norepinephrine, which is the neurotransmitter the brain uses for alertness, concentration, and long-term memory formation; and it is crucial for normal adrenal-gland function. The adrenal glands utilize more vitamin C per gram of tissue weight than any other part of the body.

Foods rich in vitamin C are broccoli, citrus fruits, strawberries, celery, kiwi, tomatoes, peppers, and cantaloupe. Vitamin C supplements are easy to find, and a reasonable dosage would be 500 mg morning and night. Nighttime supplementation of vitamin C can be especially important in recovering from an injury because the body repairs itself during sleep and utilizes vitamin C to repair connective tissue such as muscles, tendons, and ligaments.

The antioxidants known as *bioflavonoids* are so called because they occur in many of the same foods as vitamin C. Bioflavonoids are the compounds that are responsible for the color of some fruits and even flowers. Research has shown that bioflavonoids protect cell membranes, inhibit histamine release, and inhibit the dilation of the blood vessels and subsequent swelling caused by bradykinins.

While bioflavonoids occur in the same foods mentioned above for vitamin C, they are also present in rose hips, plums, cherries, black currants, eggplant, squash, parsley, and red wine. Vitamin supplements that contain both vitamin C and bioflavonoids are very easy to find, and the dosage recommendation is still predicated on a vitamin C content of 500 mg taken morning and night.

Two more very strong antioxidants are Pycnogenol and grape seed extract, which are chemically the same but come from different sources. Pycnogenol, a registered trademark, is extracted from the bark of maritime pine trees, whereas grape seed extract obviously comes from grape seeds. Since it is much easier to gain access to grape seeds, as they are a waste product of the wine industry, than it is to strip the bark off of trees, grape seed extract is less expensive.

It is estimated that grape seed extract is an antioxidant twenty times more powerful than vitamin C. This doesn't mean that you still don't need the vitamin C for connective-tissue repair, protection against infection, and support of the adrenal glands. An effective dosage of grape seed extract is 50 mg three times a day.

Other antioxidants include beta-carotene, vitamin E, and selenium. The goal of this book is not to see how many pills you can stuff into your body, however, and these can be obtained by simply taking a good-quality multiple vitamin, which I will discuss momemtarily.

THE IMPORTANCE OF PURE WATER

It is very important to note that if you are going to take antioxidants, then you must drink water throughout the day to flush the free radicals out of your body. Of course, you should be drinking water throughout the day anyway, but it becomes especially important in this case so that you don't have all of these toxins being released with no way to get out of your body.

The quality of the water that you are drinking is also very important. I personally believe that everyone needs to buy a water filter for his or her home. They come in many forms, from the inexpensive to the space age varieties that filter every faucet in the house. Even if you can't afford a thousand-dollar system, there are simple filtration devices that require nothing more than putting water into a container that has a filter in it. I don't think it's a good idea to trust our public water systems because of all the chemicals in the ground that are leaching into the water supplies. Some brands of bottled water can be suspect, as the quality varies so much, and some studies have found companies putting regular tap water into the bottles. The more expensive brands of bottled water probably live up to their claims of purity, but the cost would make drinking them on a daily basis prohibitive, and they are more appropriate for those times when you are away from home.

While distilled water is very pure and sounds like a good solution to treated and/or polluted water, there is a problem with its total lack of mineral content. Part of the value of drinking water is that it is a source of minerals. Nature abhors a vacuum, and unless your diet is exceptionally high in minerals, the distilled water is going to dilute the mineral concentration in your body. So, in the long run, it's best to buy some form of water filtration system for your home, and if you are traveling or away from home, buy a good-quality bottled water.

ORGANIC PRODUCE AND MULTIPLE VITAMINS

I would advise you to always buy organic produce whenever possible because the nutritional value is higher and you will be putting fewer toxins into your body. It doesn't make sense to consume produce that has been sprayed with all kinds of chemicals and then take antioxidant pills to try to get the chemicals out of your body.

There used to be some debate as to whether you can really get all of the essential nutrients from your diet given the way food is grown and produced these days, but very recently the American Medical Association (AMA), which up until now has generally scoffed at vitamins and nutritional therapies, put an end to this debate when it issued an advisory recommending that everyone should take a multiple vitamin on a daily basis. A good approach is to find a really good-quality multiple vitamin and mineral supplement in a health food or vitamin store and take it every day. While it is still essential that you have a well-balanced diet, this should fill in any nutritional gaps that might exist.

By adopting a commonsense approach to the foods you choose to eat, understanding your relationship with food, and making a commitment to treat your body with the respect it deserves, you will lose weight (if you need to) and feel so much better by having the proper fuel your body requires to function at its optimal level.

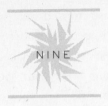

NINE

PSYCHOLOGICAL STRESS

"It's all in your mind, you know."
—GEORGE HARRISON

lthough the focus of this book is primarily on the relationship between the physiological stressors of pain, intestinal-tract and systemic inflammation, and imbalanced cortisol levels, it is important that we discuss the role of psychological stress as well. Acute psychological stress will raise cortisol levels just as much as physical pain and inflammation, and if it becomes chronic, it can eventually lead to adrenal-gland burnout and cortisol depletion.

Of equal importance is the fact that, for some people, chronic psychological stress can cause intestinal-tract irritation and inflammation and thus perpetuate the physiological-stress scenarios discussed in the previous chapter. Keeping in mind that each person's body can respond to stress differently, elevated levels of cortisol in some people will inhibit the normal tissue repair necessary for the digestive tract to counterbalance the daily onslaught caused by the routine caustic acids required for digesting food. The progressive inflammation caused by the acids will then further elevate the cortisol levels, and we are back to the vicious cycle of interplay between the two types of stress: physiological and psychological.

For most people, "I'm so stressed-out" is the catch phrase that defines their lives. According to people's daily conversations, the prevalence of stress in their lives appears to have reached epidemic proportions. It comes from your job, your boss, your spouse or significant other, your kids, your parents, your siblings, your computer, your television, your newspaper, other drivers, and most of all, the guy in the nine-items-or-less cash-only express checkout line at the grocery store with fifteen items and his checkbook. It seems like everyone is stressed-out about something these days, and stress is a major focal point of many a discussion.

THE SUBJECTIVE PERCEPTION OF STRESS

The single most intriguing aspect of psychological stress is that it is almost completely subjective. I think most people would initially disagree with this because we all harbor the illusion that our reactions to our stressors are "normal" and "correct," e.g., the old "who wouldn't be angry/mad/upset" in response to a certain set of circumstances. There is also a list of the top ten stressors considered to be universal, such as the death of a loved one, the loss of employment, divorce, and so on.

However, consider the divorce in which one person doesn't want the dissolution of the marriage and will be left broken-hearted and burdened with the role of single parent, while the other person will be embarking on a romantic adventure with a new partner. Or maybe the spouse who is being left behind to be the single parent is thrilled to see the abusive lout finally leave.

Another example of the subjectivity of the stress response would be the death of a loved one, the obvious response to which would be intense grief. However, if the circumstances of this loved one's death involved horrible prolonged suffering from the ravages of cancer, then the emotional response might be one of relief that the person's pain has ended, and the grief might be a good deal less. Allowing for different cultural perspectives, some societies view death as a joyous occasion when the loved one is passing on to a far better place, and so there is no need to mourn his or her departure. It's all a matter of what you believe to be true.

The famous philosopher J. Krishnamurti would often take questions from audiences following his lectures. His most common response to all of these very sincere questions, which were usually concerned with the disharmony among people, how peace could be found, the meaning of life, or the nature of love, was "Why do you think that?" This response would usually cause the person asking the question to try to rephrase it, as if Krishnamurti didn't understand the original one. But after hearing it a second time, Krishnamurti would simply ask again, "Why do you think that?" What he was doing was challenging the rules and beliefs about life and the thinking process that led his listeners to their assumptions and conclusions regarding the human condition. He was asking them to look inside their minds and to follow the constructs that, to them, seemed to form their own brand of "logical, rational thought" and to see, truly, where that idea came from. Krishnamurti had a great awareness and understanding of the subjectivity of human thought and behavior as well as the problems it can cause.

TAKING CONTROL OF WHAT YOU THINK AND FEEL

How we respond to any given psychological stress is entirely up to us, which by itself is a huge problem. It takes an enormous degree of character to choose to be responsible for all that occurs in your life and to realize that even if you can't control all of the events, you *can* control how you feel about it.

If you decide that no one or nothing can make you feel anything other than what you choose, then you are in possession of great personal power. But it also means that you will have to develop the habit of paying attention to *what* you are thinking and the *why* of it. It is easier to blame other people or circumstances for your anger, disappointment, sadness, and failures than to make yourself responsible. It is more tempting to believe something your parents, teachers, or friends told you about how to think or feel or to go with the flow of popular opinion rather than have to examine the thought process by which you determine what makes you happy or angry. But like it or not, you are the one who chooses your responses, either actively or passively, and the more you accept that fact, the more control you will have over what you perceive to be stressful.

There is an old saying that opinions are like rectums, everybody's got one. While the latter serves a useful function, the former often does not. Think for a bit about your day and the internal dialogue you have had with yourself. You know, that wonderful little voice inside your head that either makes you take note of what a beautiful day it is or the one that whines and moans endlessly about other people's lifestyles, clothing, driving skills, behavior toward you or others, and on and on. A great question to ask yourself at times when you are on a negative roll is "Why do I have to have an opinion about this?" Why indeed. What possible good can come from focusing on a litany of negativity as a response to your environment and the people who inhabit it?

People often get trapped in a negative-thinking mode. I think part of the problem is that it is fundamental to existence to regard everything we encounter with a survivalist view, asking first "Does this present any danger to me?" It is, in fact, how our sensory nervous system works and how we perceive stress. All of our sensory information, be it sight, sound, taste, smell, or touch, is first neurologically perceived by the limbic system in our brains, which is where our survivalist stress center originates. It is the job of the limbic system to assess the stimulus, decide if it presents a danger to the body, and then initiate the appropriate reaction. If you touch something that is too hot, your limbic system will cause your muscles to contract and move you away from the heat. The limbic system is always evaluating everything that is happening, like a watchful guard dog.

The problem here is that when there is not much to guard against, when you are safe from harm and on automatic pilot, your brain just can't be still. We create a lot of mental dialogue over nothing because we have not learned how to allow our minds to be still and because the limbic system is attuned to watching out for negative, dangerous events. We let that little voice inside run rampant as it engages in endless, and mostly useless, monologues in which we just seem to need to have one opinion after another. I think many people learn to look for the negative rather than to focus on the positive and think they are doing themselves a favor in a Boy Scout–like effort to "be prepared." A recent research study reports that even in times of prosperity and safety, people still worry a lot and suffer anxiety concerning their future. It is this kind of thought process that gives life to Murphy's Law: the expectation that whatever can go wrong will go wrong.

A better approach to dealing with this mental dialogue is first to be aware of it on a conscious level and not just let it run off on its own and then to be less judgmental about every little thing. This can be very liberating and at times funny when you catch yourself wasting your time and energy wondering why in the world that teenager's pants are hanging down so low (answer: he is practicing to be a future plumber) or any number of silly things we choose to have an opinion about and clog up our brains with on a daily basis.

This approach of asking yourself why you have to have an opinion about everything gives you an immediately empowering example of how you can actively choose your responses instead of allowing your mind to jabber away. Another benefit you will derive is a sense of less pressure on yourself, for judgment implies standards, your own in this case, that you are using to measure yourself against other people. In the Bible it says, "Judge not, lest ye be judged." By not being so consumed with comparing yourself to everyone else, you can be more relaxed and accepting of yourself and maintain an attitude of live and let live.

PSYCHOLOGICAL FACTORS OF STRESS

In his extraordinary book, *Why Zebras Don't Get Ulcers,* Dr. Robert Sapolsky discusses numerous research studies on the psychological factors of stress. What appear to be the two most important components in the response to this type of stress are control and predictability. The amount of control and predictability a human or research animal has, or even perceives it has, greatly determines what effect the stress will have on him or her. A rat that has some means of controlling the frequency of electric shocks will get fewer ulcers than a rat that has no control. Similarly, a rat that is warned when the shocks will occur will have a stress response that is less intense than that of the rat given no warning. At some point, if it is shocked frequently enough, the rat will perceive the shock as a predictable stressor and again will have a weaker stress response. A rat that has been trained to use a lever to avoid shocks will have a massive stress response if the lever is taken away, and the stress response will weaken if the lever is returned, even if it is disconnected and doesn't actually prevent the shock from occurring. Just believing that it has some means of control helps the rat reduce its stress levels.

The negative effects of stress and the issue of control apply equally to humans. A recent four-year study conducted by the Harvard Center for Society and Health assessed the effects of job stress on 21,000 women. It was found that a stressful job can cause as much wear and tear on the body as smoking and that the women in the study who experienced the most job strain also experienced the most health problems. These women were at greater risk for hypertension or high blood pressure as well as for an increased general rate of illness; some even had difficulty walking, climbing stairs, or carrying out their daily activities. This correlates well with my initial assertion that imbalanced levels of cortisol can lead to high blood pressure, immune-system dysfunction, and fatigue. What this study also found was that the women who had some control over their schedules and duties were less affected by the stress of their jobs.

It would seem logical that we all want some level of control over the things that occur in our lives and some degree of predictability of events. The problem again comes back to just how much responsibility we want to assume in making our lives as stress-free as possible.

The often incongruous opinions and judgments that make up our thoughts and actions get us into all kinds of trouble. When I was a freshman in college, I had a history professor who began and ended every class with the statement "It's not what *is* that counts, it's what people *think* that counts." Throughout the entire history course he would prove this point over and over again by illustrating how wars were waged and people were slaughtered wholesale on the basis of a belief or a perception of what was "real." How we decide what is stressful to us goes right back to our own perception of what is happening to us and how that perception coincides with our opinions and judgments.

The best technique I know of for dealing with psychological stress is to take control and examine your thought process. Sit yourself down with paper and pen and write down exactly *what* it is you feel stressed about, then write down *why* you feel stressed about it. In most cases, what will ultimately come to the surface is a discrepancy between your opinions and judgments about how your life should be and your perceptions of how it is, or a discrepancy between your opinions and judgments and those of someone else, with stress being the end result of your reaction to the discrepancy. This would then be a good time to really look at your opinions and judgments and to see just exactly where they came from and how much conscious effort went into making them. Do they really make sense and are they reasonable, or are they just a bundle of immature wishes and desires thrown together?

This is a process that can take some time, so don't expect to sit down and get your life and all of its stresses worked out in twenty minutes. It also requires some insight and honesty. It can provoke many emotions and at times can even be a little painful because people do not like to admit that they, or what they are thinking, are wrong. But if your opinions and judgments about life are burning up your adrenal glands, then it is better to come to terms with them now before they give you a heart attack or an ulcer.

A compulsive necessity to be "right" in one's opinions or judgments can cause an enormous amount of pain, both emotional and physical. In my quarter century of clinical practice, I have observed numerous cases in which the primary cause of a patient's physical pain was due to an opinion, and the pain was absolutely necessary in order to make that opinion "right." One example would be that of an employee who harbored the belief that his employer was mean, overbearing, and determined to work people to death, and who consequently developed a pain syndrome that "proved" the destructive intentions of the employer. No amount of treatment would relieve this person's pain because if the pain was resolved and he was still working for the same employer, then his opinion about his employer would turn out to be "wrong," and that would have been completely unacceptable.

OUR OPINIONS AND JUDGMENTS

Our opinions and judgments in the game of life are actually not hard to understand; they begin as exercises in conditioned response administered by our parents, siblings, schoolmates, teachers, the media, and so on. When we are very young we learn these rules through trial and error, as our reasoning skills are not yet very well developed. It is impossible for an infant to reason that throwing a bowl of baby food across the room is inappropriate because of the mess it will make and the extra work it will bring to her parent's already hectic day. So the unreasoning kid will launch the bowl with much glee, only to find her future in aerodynamic research stunted by some immediate form of reprimand or punishment. At this point in her early life, this child does not have a thought-out strategy for managing her response to this stressful experience and will probably start crying.

As we get older we experience a lot more of this cause-and-effect business but with help from our reasoning minds, minds that can project the consequences of causing a big mess and thus prevent us from taking the action. So far so good, except that the people who are helping us form our opinions may have some very irrational opinions of their own that they are passing on. Unfortunately, there is nothing that can be done about this, although I personally favor the dog-child rule, which is that before you are allowed to have a kid, you have to get a dog. If you can successfully train the dog, then you get to have a kid. Nevertheless, as we get older, we continue to acquire our opinions and judgments through our experiences and interactions with all manner of people and stimuli.

At some point I think all of us arrive at a place where we begin to question what's going on in our heads (parents know this as adolescence), and we make an effort to determine if what we have been taught to think and feel is valid. But just how committed we are to evaluate this in depth and on an ongoing basis will greatly affect our ability to manage our emotions, behavior, and responses to stress. If you are being conditioned by a bad parent or teacher to believe that you are stupid, lazy, worthless, and won't amount to anything of value, you are doomed—unless you take it upon yourself to question and challenge these assumptions. People who survive adverse childhood conditions of abuse, poverty, and violence do so by making their own evaluations of these situations and adopting rules and beliefs that defy their circumstances.

I am not suggesting a micromanagement approach to evaluating every thought or feeling you have, because that will lead to obsessive-compulsive behavior, and then you will be plenty stressed out. What would be more appropriate would be to do an initial checkup on yourself, looking at the more significant opinions and judgments you have now, and to see if they make sense and enhance your life. For example, harboring an opinion/judgment that for me to be happy I absolutely must be a multimillionaire living in Tahiti while dating the Swedish women's volleyball team is probably not going to make for a stress-free existence. On the other hand, if I construct my life around opinions and judgments that enable me to be a positive influence on other people's lives, making every day count, having goals to achieve, and counting my blessings, then it is going to be a lot easier to be content at the end of each day. If I insist on having opinions that are immature, unrealistic, or incongruent, then I am setting myself up for failure and disappointment.

BEING IN CHARGE OF YOUR LIFE

Most people spend more time planning their annual two-week vacation than they do planning the rest of their lives. They wake up and basically let the day happen to them rather than start out with a proactive concept of what they want the day to be like, what they want to accomplish, and what kind of relationship they want to have with the people they will encounter.

Every day people drag themselves off to work with no better chance of things going consistently well than if they were to get in a boat with no compass and push off the dock in the hope they will land in Tahiti. Since Dr. Sapolsky's research clearly shows that the two major components of psychological stress are control and predictability of events, it makes a great deal of sense to begin each day by having at least a concept or "prediction" of what you wish to have happen. Obviously not everything may go as planned, but at least you are starting out with some sense of control, and as long as you don't have a rule that says everything must go as planned or you will shoot yourself, you will probably feel less stressed-out. Remember that the rat that believes it has control even if the lever that would prevent the shock doesn't work still has a less intense response to stress. So how hard would it be to take a few minutes at the beginning of each day to think about what kind of day you wish to have in order to gain a sense of control over your life, or to decide that nothing is going to make you angry or upset and that you—not someone else—will choose how you feel or that you don't have to have an opinion about every little thing you see or hear.

Another example of taking control is looking at your attitude when you arrive home from work each day. Do you take a moment to compose yourself and actively think about what kind of relationship you want to have with your spouse, kids, or whomever, or do you just leap out of the car, bound through the door, and see what happens next? How much control and predictability is involved in that? Or do you expect to be treated a certain way because you worked hard today, without considering that the other people in your life have their own expectations and that these might not be totally compatible with yours? Again, the more you become aware of how and what you are thinking and the more you are consciously directing your life, the less stress you will encounter.

Taking Action

With any technique designed to help manage psychological stress success depends on action, meaning that you can read about stress reduction all day long and understand the concept very well, but until you actually *do* something to change your stress response, nothing is really going to change. This is where some stress-management techniques run into trouble: Because they are too time consuming, they end up as just another stressor.

The activities I am recommending are easy and don't take much time; in fact, they have been designed to be done in small increments to ensure success. The following activities do not have to be done in any particular order, so just start with the ones that seem the easiest and most comfortable to do, but plan to be doing all of them at some point, and *don't quit*. Since it is easier to learn a new habit when it is linked with something you are already doing on a daily basis, the following list follows this approach.

- Give yourself five extra minutes before you get out of bed in the morning to reflect on what kind of day you want to have; what objectives you want to achieve; what kinds of emotions you want to experience. If you were a movie director going to the set to film today's scene of *Your Life*, what would the movie look like at the end of the day's shooting?
- When you are taking your shower or bath, don't let your mind get filled up with a bunch of gibberish, but be fully present and *feel* the physical sensation of the hot water, the

smell of the soap, and the massaging of the shampoo in your hair. Then take a moment to realize how lucky you are to have indoor plumbing, hot water, and a functional bathroom, which millions of people throughout the world do not have.

- Every time before you eat, take fifteen seconds (or longer if you wish) to be grateful for actually having something to eat, and remember that not everyone in this world is so fortunate.

- If you are in a relationship with a "significant other," find a reason or an opportunity every day to tell that person that you love him or her. Life is short, and you don't want to regret missing any chance to bring happiness into your lover's life.

- Whether or not you are romantically involved with someone, you are still in a relationship with the world around you. On your way to and from work or while running errands, turn down the mental noise in your head and turn up your senses, paying attention to the sights and sounds around you. Noticing the incredible natural beauty of the world you live in also has the reciprocal effect of turning down that mental noise, so the more aware you are, the less stressed-out you will be.

- In addition to the relationship you may have with a lover or with the physical world in which you exist, there is your relationship with and interdependence on a myriad of people who directly impact your life and make it "work." I very much enjoy being a doctor and love my job, but I am acutely aware that without my office staff, the grocery clerk, my waste-disposal service, my car mechanic, and a whole host of other people and the services they provide for me, my life would be far more difficult. You come into contact with these people on a daily basis. Be appreciative of all of the people who affect your life and show them your appreciation.

- Beyond all of these external relationships is the one you have with yourself. Each day find a reason to tell yourself that you love you, because of a good deed you have done, because you accomplished what you set out to do, or simply because you found some enjoyment in that particular day. Taking a few minutes before going to sleep to reflect upon your day and how you lived it is a good way to end your day.

- Get a good old-fashioned paper calendar that has each month on a separate page. At the beginning of each month, on a separate piece of paper, write down a list of five things you are currently worried about. Then take that list and tape it to the next month's page. At the end of the month when you turn to the next month's page and find your list, see how important those worries were, or if they even still exist, since you have possibly come up with a whole new list of worries. This is a good way to gain some perspective on what we think is stressful and on how transitory these worries can be. Of course, if you are dealing with your own serious illness or that of a loved one, an extended period of unemployment, or your burned-down house, then the stress may certainly extend into the next month. But, by and large, you will come to realize that many of the things you worried about weren't worth the bother in the first place.

HORMONE IMBALANCE AND RATIONAL THINKING

There is no doubt that having a clearer understanding of what your opinions and judgments really are, seeing how they are impacting your life on a daily basis, deciding to take charge of your life, and then implementing a positive plan of action that enables you to manage stress more effectively by giving you a greater sense of control and predictability will enhance the quality of your life. Learning to handle psychological stress better is certainly important, because not doing so is going to result in elevated levels of cortisol and a myriad of related physical problems.

However, this is a good place to come to terms with the fact that if your cortisol levels are already chronically elevated due to physical inflammation that may be the result of prolonged psychological stress and its effect on the intestinal tract or to the overuse of NSAIDs, antibiotics, or a pro-inflammatory diet, then it is entirely possible that the cortisol imbalance will impede your ability to cope with psychological stress. It's the vicious cycle again.

Numerous researchers have documented that the nerve cells in our brains can be ravaged by elevated levels of cortisol, especially in the hippocampus and amygdala. As you will recall from Chapter 2, these two parts of the limbic system make perceptual judgments about incoming information. Our ability to make rational sense of our world is dependent on how well these nerve cells work, and elevated levels of cortisol can impair their function.

This is why, if you have the symptoms I have thus far been describing, it is so important to have your cortisol levels tested. It will prove to be very difficult for you to rationally assess the quality of your opinions and judgments, or to do well in any of the other areas of psychological stress management that we have been discussing, if your cortisol levels are impairing the parts of the brain you use to make these judgments.

So now it is time to move on to learning all about the method and meaning of salivary cortisol testing.

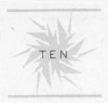

THE EMOTIONAL
COMPONENT OF ILLNESS

An Elusive Roadblock
to Regaining Good Health

ongratulations, you have conquered your pain syndrome, you have repaired your intestinal lining, and your cortisol/DHEA ratios are normal. But you still don't feel too spunky? If that's the case, it is now time to come full circle from the discussion of psychological stress in Chapter 9 to the emotional component of illness.

Not everyone who has a pain syndrome or a chronic illness will necessarily have this emotional component, and of those who do, some cases may be much more complicated than others. It is easy to understand why people who are having a lot of pain that is limiting their lifestyle and interrupting their sleep might be depressed or irritable. And if in addition to a pain-inducing structural disorder, they also suffer from the chemical component of leaky-gut syndrome and cortisol imbalances, it's all that much easier to understand why they don't feel well emotionally. For many people, all it takes is the resolution of their structural and chemical problems to restore them physically and mentally to their usual selves.

Unfortunately, some people get their physical problems resolved but continue to not thrive. Either their problems transform into some new complaint, or the old ones have a nasty way of recurring. In these cases, the emotional component of illness must be explored.

The Three Factors of the Emotional Component

In my experience treating patients, there are usually three factors at play in the emotional arena. The first has to do with something known as *learned helplessness;* the second is control-coping skills; and the last factor is subconscious conditioned-response triggers. These factors can occur separately or in combination.

Learned Helplessness

Learned helplessness is a term used to describe an animal that has been conditioned in such a way that it can no longer cope appropriately with even the most mundane tasks in its life. In laboratory experiments, two psychologists, Martin Seligman and Steven Maier, exposed two groups of rats to huge amounts of stress and then tested the effects of control and predictability on how the rats would respond to the stress.

The first group of rats was trained in what is known as an *active-avoidance task.* This was accomplished by putting a rat in a cage where half of the floor would transmit an electrical shock and where, prior to giving the shock, the rat would be given a signal indicating which side of the floor would become electrified. Once it had learned the signal, the rat would reliably move to the side of the cage that would not transmit the shock. These rats did not show any increased signs of stress because they had learned how to control their situation.

The second group of rats was exposed to frequent electrical shocks and noise over a long period of time with no warning, no ability to control the stimuli, and no sense of predictability as to when they would occur. These rats exhibited many of the same characteristics seen in human depression: elevated cortisol levels, disturbed sleep cycles, and a loss of motivation. These rats were then placed in the same environment as the first group of rats, where signals and warnings were given before the shocks, and were *unable* to learn the active-avoidance task. Even attempts to reward the rats beyond enabling them to avoid the shocks, such as giving them food or sex, failed to change their behavior. It seems that once the rats were conditioned into learned helplessness, embracing the perception that there was nothing they could do to change or improve their situation, they were permanently damaged in their ability to cope even when the dynamics of their situation changed.

Learned helplessness has been demonstrated in studies using dogs, cats, birds, and humans. There are frightening and insidious implications in how easily some human beings can be conditioned into learned helplessness. Going back to one of the most basic premises of this book, each individual responds differently to stress, which is a very fortunate thing. Unfortunately, there are studies on underprivileged children that show that their overall inability to read was a result of their being conditioned to believe that they were intellectually incapable of the task.

Let's take a look at how learned helplessness can become a factor in a pain syndrome or chronic illness. You will recall that Dr. Robert Sapolsky, the Stanford University stress researcher, states that the two greatest psychological stressors are the lack of control and lack of predictability.

So there you are, with a chronic pain syndrome, leaky-gut, systemic inflammation, and you feel like your body is sabotaging you. Sometimes you hurt, sometimes you don't; the pain wanders around, and the degree of pain varies from tolerable to intolerable. Some nights you sleep, and some nights you are wide awake staring at the ceiling. Some days you are tense and irritable, and other days you are so lethargic you can barely move. You don't understand what in the world is wrong with you, and your loved ones are beginning to wonder about you as well.

It seems that you have no control over how you are going to feel from one day to the next nor can you predict which activities you may or may not engage in. This is when the emotional stress adds to the stress you already have from physical pain and gastrointestinal inflammation and when your adrenal glands' ability to manage the stress is progressively declining.

Now logic would suggest that after resolving the structural pain syndrome and the chemical cortisol imbalance, your emotional life would just go back to normal. But as we have seen with the experiments on learned helplessness, that is not always the case. For some people who have experienced chronic or repetitive episodes of pain or long-term cortisol imbalances, learned helplessness insidiously becomes part of their personality.

The prolonged pain and/or cortisol imbalance changes their external perception of the world around them and their internal perception of their ability to cope with that world. They become fearful of activity because they think it might produce pain, and they don't allow themselves to do things that were once a source of fun. They no longer go skiing or dancing, and they avoid long trips because they are afraid that these activities will cause a recurrence of pain.

They become socially withdrawn because they are used to being anxious, depressed, or both, and don't feel very comfortable around other people. They have learned not to trust their bodies and are waiting for the next bad thing to happen, as it always has in the past. Even when they are not in any pain and there is no intestinal inflammation causing an elevation of cortisol, they continue to sleep poorly because they go to bed worrying if it will be a good night or a bad night, and the worrying raises cortisol levels to the point where they cause insomnia.

This brings us to the mind/body research study being done at the University of Iowa, where they are using brain scans that measure blood flow to different parts of the brain while the test subjects are thinking of specific emotions. What this study has revealed is that certain emotions will influence neurological activity in parts of the brain that are also associated with muscle and organ function. So what may be happening in learned helplessness with regard to illness is a case of self-fulfilling prophecy, meaning that the constant worry or expectation of bad things occurring causes a negative neurological stimulus in the part of the brain that will actually cause these bad things to happen. This just reaffirms the helplessness, and the cycle continues.

Control-Coping Skills

The second factor in the emotional component of illness is the control-coping skill, which is a kind of bizarre twist on learned helplessness. It involves using the illness to gain control and predictability of one's life. In most cases, I think this starts out innocently enough as a fair response to being in pain or being ill, but over time it takes on a life of its own and grows from being subconscious to subtly intentional.

This factor has its origin in childhood, when we discover that we can stay home from school and get lots of attention if we become ill. That works well until one day we realize that we forgot to do a book report or study for a test, and we fake being sick to get out of going to school. Since our parents surely tried this trick on their parents, they are not so easily fooled, and you end up suffering the double whammy of having to go to school unprepared along with the punishment you will receive when you get home for trying to pull such a stunt. This is usually enough to teach us to not make a career out of being "sick."

However, some people learn a very different lesson about being ill. What they learn is that because they are ill, the people around them are sympathetic and give them more attention. They also can't be expected to clean the house, do the dishes, mow the lawn, or seek gainful employment. Should the people around them begin to complain about their prolonged illness, they are only going to get sicker from the additional stress, and God knows we wouldn't want that to happen. The person who is ill now gets to decide if and when certain activities take place, like going on trips or going to a movie and which movie it will be, lest he has to sit too long or watch something that might upset him, or if there might be sex that night and in just what position, and the list goes on and on.

This is not to say that these people don't have some or all of the physical problems I have previously discussed regarding pain syndromes, intestinal-tract and/or systemic inflammation, and cortisol imbalances. It's just that they have learned to use their illnesses to control virtually every aspect of their lives either consciously or subconsciously. The world revolves around them, and all decisions regarding family, friends, employment, and activities are regulated by how they feel.

To make matters worse, look at what they will lose should they ever get well. Their entire lives will change in ways they may perceive as not particularly desirable. The idea of having to return to being a regular person whose needs do not supersede anyone else's after months or, more typically, years of being in control and being relieved of many responsibilities, can be frightening. The concept of going back to work, being socially engaged, and having additional responsibilities after years of dealing with pain and stress-related disorders, can seem overwhelming and, of course, very stressful. So while their physical conditions might improve over time, they never really get well and linger at some plateau that enables them to remain in control.

One aspect of control-coping skill and how it relates to learned helplessness is that these people decide that certain activities are the cause of their problems and, therefore, must be avoided forever. For example, if you are suffering from lower-back pain, which is frequently caused by activities that require bending forward, you might perceive vacuuming the carpet as a very risky task. Even if you recover from the back pain, you might decide that you must never vacuum again because you consider it a causative factor. The fact that you can vacuum a rug without bending forward by just pushing the upright vacuum cleaner while standing up straight has never occurred to you. But, most important, as a control-coping skill you have found a way to get someone else to do the vacuuming.

As the person gains more control, she can arrive at the conclusion that she pretty much can't do *anything* without getting into trouble, so she decides that it is better to do nothing and to have other people perform these physical tasks. A more appropriate response would be to learn to do these activities using proper bending and lifting techniques (always bend from the knees, not from the waist) and to consult a physical therapist or personal trainer in order to get into better physical shape.

All of this, however, brings us back to the fear or dread of the trappings of a "normal" life and the perceived stress inherent in being well and not having any valid reasons for being excused from the everyday responsibilities that affect most people.

When I encounter this behavior in patients, I find it important not to criticize the person but to make them aware of it. This is not hypochondria or a psychological disorder; this is a coping skill that they have learned in the face of chronic pain and hormonal imbalance. In the example I gave earlier about hormones overriding rational thought concerning whether or not to eat a candy bar, you will recall that the hormonally induced craving always wins; this is the same thing. Even though patients may be responding well to treatment, the fear they associate with their condition and activity can still cause an elevation of cortisol, which keeps them going around in circles. While the logical part of their brains rationally concludes that being healthy is a desirable thing, the hormonal chemicals in their brains induce a fear that is hard to overcome.

By making patients aware of this syndrome, they can begin to realize more clearly what their fears are and how they may be sabotaging their efforts to get well. I find it useful to have them go home and write down five positive and five negative changes that would occur in their lives if they were completely healthy. As you might imagine, some patients get defensive and declare that there are no negative aspects to their getting well, but when I ask them when was the last time they cleaned the house, mowed the lawn, raked the leaves, took out the garbage, washed the car, and so on, they get the idea.

I also challenge them to reevaluate why they think that being healthy will mean that they have to change their lives in a way they associate with stress. After all, if they haven't been doing these tasks for months or years, why do they assume that they will have to do so now? Obviously these responsibilities are being managed in some other way, and perhaps there is no reason for them to feel that an overwhelming wave of new obligations will come crashing down on them simply because they are no longer physically impaired.

It is also very important to remind them that just because they have had problems in the past, it does not mean they are destined to have them in the future. By achieving success in a good treatment program, by learning the correct biomechanics of how to use their bodies to avoid reinjury, and by having their hormonal imbalances resolved, they will be living their lives on a different playing field. They will have gained the knowledge of what went wrong and know that not only can it be corrected, it also can be prevented from recurring. Knowledge is a powerful tool.

Subconscious Conditioned-Response Triggers

This brings us to the third factor in the emotional component of getting well: subconscious conditioned-response triggers. Even after resolving their pain syndromes and hormonal imbalances, and armed with the strategies for dealing successfully with their health, sometimes patients cannot align themselves with their thoughts and emotions. They understand their health issues intellectually, but they simply cannot get past their conditioned responses. These subconscious triggers often play a significant role in the learned helplessness and control-coping skills components.

As it pertains to learned helplessness, patients who have successfully recovered from their pain syndromes and/or cortisol imbalances understand intellectually that they should be able to lift objects or to garden without ending up in pain, or that they should be able to sleep or to encounter social situations without unnecessary anxieties. However, they are not "emotionally congruent," and the mere sight of a wheelbarrow or the thought of being involved in a situation that used to cause pain or anxiety triggers a fear response that prevents them from properly adapting to the situation.

The control-coping–skills component is equally vulnerable to subconscious triggers. While people who are using a physical disorder as a means of controlling their environment are busy assuring themselves and those around them that they really want to get well, they are emotionally incongruent with the concept of being well and losing control.

A good example of this is Ivan Pavlov and his hallmark research with dogs and conditioned responses. By consistently ringing a bell before feeding the dogs, he conditioned the dogs to associate food with the bell and to salivate when they heard the bell. Even when he stopped feeding them after ringing the bell, the dogs continued to salivate when the bell rang.

The same process occurs in the human model, where you know intellectually that there is no reason to metaphorically "salivate" just because you hear the "bell," but your conditioning is so strong that you do it anyway. For human beings, it does not require repetitive reinforcement to anchor the conditioning; often the conditioning is the result of an emotionally charged moment. The problem is, during a highly charged emotional event, the perception of what is happening and the meaning that the brain attaches to it may not be completely rooted in reality. Nevertheless, these events get stored in our memory banks and can be triggered by other sensory stimuli that might have been circumstantially present when the original event occurred.

Events make a biochemical impression on the brain, specifically in the hippocampus, which, as previously discussed, deals with short-term memory. To file experiences away permanently, the hippocampus shunts the elements of the experience—the sounds, smells, sights—through a network of nerve cells to different areas of the brain. "It's a whole cascade of processes, physiological and chemical, that sensitizes the neurons to transmit messages," notes Mortimer Mishkin, chief of the neuropsychology laboratory of the National Institutes of Health. The proper stimulus—say, a whiff of perfume or a glimpse of a familiar place—trips the relay, firing the neurons and bringing a past event into consciousness.

A great way to test this is to turn on the radio to what would be an "oldies" station relative to your age group and see how different songs trigger memories of where you were at that time, the friends you had, and even of a particular girlfriend or boyfriend. Some songs will seem like the theme of an entire summer or will remind you of your first kiss or the times you drove around with your friends with hardly a care in the world. Or pull out that shoe box of pictures collecting dust under your bed and see how looking at them brings up memories of the people and events that were taking place when the pictures were snapped. After all, isn't that the whole purpose of taking pictures in the first place?

The downside of this is that a stimulus can also trigger an unconscious response of an emotionally negative experience, which then neurologically inhibits the normal function of an organ or muscle group (referring back to the research at the University of Iowa that shows the association of emotions linked to the parts of the brain that relate to specific organs and muscles). Tragically, childhood victims of physical or sexual abuse are prone to these responses. The San Francisco Spine Institute, which deals with patients with complicated and serious spinal disorders, has found that there is a higher incidence of chronic back pain in people who have suffered such childhood abuse. One possible reason for this may be the conditioned response of tightening the lower-back muscles to arch back in an attempt to elude an attack. But what happens when these people, as adults, encounter a sensory stimulus that unconsciously triggers a memory of an attack? Suppose they go to the grocery store and encounter a perfume or cologne that smells like that of their attacker, and then, as they bend to put their groceries in the car, their back goes into a spasm. In the course of their lifetime they may have put hundreds of bags of groceries into their vehicle with no problem, but in this instance their back muscles were emotionally induced into a state of tension, and then just a small physical movement evoked a complete spasm.

EMOTIONAL STRESS AND NECK AND LOWER-BACK PAIN

There appears to be a high correlation between stress and neck and lower-back pain, and while there is definitive research that shows that *all* primates will tense their trapezius muscles (those great big muscles that attach the neck to the shoulders and that you love to have massaged) when stressed or angered, no one knows why. After twenty-five years of practice and thinking about this, my clinical hunch is that there is a neurological connection between the nerves of the neck and lower back and the adrenal glands.

There is a group of nerves that emerges from the vertebrae of the neck, called the *brachial plexus,* which comprises the entire nerve supply of the upper limbs. Similarly, the group of nerves exiting the vertebrae of the lower back forms the *lumbo-sacral plexus,* which furnishes the entire nerve supply to the lower limbs. The human response to stress is often referred to as the *fight-or-flight syndrome,* which implies that you are going to resolve a physically threatening situation by using either your arm muscles for fighting or your leg muscles for fleeing to safety or some combination of both. Since the adrenal glands orchestrate this response, it is highly probable that cortisol stimulates the function of these neurological plexuses to carry out the muscular functions necessary to survive the stress.

This response to stress and the firing of these neurological plexuses are great if you're wrestling an alligator or being chased by a mountain lion. But if the stress is psychological or the cortisol level is elevated by inflammation and the arm and leg muscles are not involved in fighting or fleeing, then activating the nerve plexuses of the neck and lower back is probably a prescription for pain and nothing more. It is very common for people to say that they hold their stress in their neck and upper back muscles (the trapezius muscles), and the statement is neurologically correct. We also seem to know intuitively that stress affects these areas, as we frequently refer to stressful situations or people as being a pain in the neck or a pain in the ass.

In many of these instances the stress is transitory, and the muscles relax, returning to their prestress status. However, should the stress be prolonged or related to a highly charged emotional event, then the muscles may remain fixated, restrict the ability of the spinal joints to move normally, and result in joint dysfunction and pain. If the stress response is triggered by an emotional event, then this syndrome can go on forever, and patients may not understand why they keep having problems.

RESOLVING CONDITIONED-RESPONSE TRIGGERS

Fortunately, there is a treatment technique that addresses these negative emotionally charged conditioned responses that interfere with normal physical function, and it is called *neuro-emotional technique (NET)*. This technique, created by Dr. Scott Walker, a chiropractor from Encinitas, California, is based on the current research regarding neuropeptides, which are the chemicals that transmit emotions.

Dr. Walker's work embraces the reality that emotional events can get locked into different parts of our bodies, and he terms these events *neuro-emotional complexes* (NECs). Furthermore, he states that not all NECs correspond with actual or historical reality, as they may be the result of perceptual misconceptions, and so he views NECs as the patient's emotional reality. It is this reality that the patient experienced and remembers, proving once again that most of life, and stress, is perceptual.

Neuro-emotional technique is a methodology used to normalize negative physical and/or behavioral patterns that have become locked into the body. Just as the researchers from the University of Iowa are seeing the neurological correlation between emotions and organ/muscle function, NET makes these same connections and assists in eliminating these negative patterns.

Dr. Elmer Green, the Mayo Clinic physician who pioneered biofeedback as a treatment for disease, has stated, "Every change in the physiological state is accompanied by an appropriate change in the mental emotional state, conscious or unconscious, and conversely, every change in the mental emotional state, conscious or unconscious, is accompanied by an appropriate change in the physiological state."

Candace B. Pert, Ph.D., was one of the leading researchers at the National Institutes of Health in a study to find opiate receptors in the brain, which led to the discovery of endorphins (our own naturally produced pain-relieving chemicals) and the subsequent mapping of the brain's neurotransmitter receptor sites. In her book, *Molecules of Emotion*, she describes in detail the body-mind relationship between the neurotransmitter chemicals of emotions and somatic, or physical, function. She goes on to say: "Most psychologists treat the mind as disembodied, a phenomenon with little or no connection to the physical body. Conversely, physicians treat the body with little or no regard to the mind or the emotions. But the body and mind are not separate, and we cannot treat one without the other. My research has shown me that the body can and must be healed through the mind, and the mind can and must be healed through the body." Dr. Pert is currently engaged in a research project with Dr. Walker that seeks further applications of the neuro-emotional technique to correct mind/body imbalances.

The Wedding Bell Blues

One example of how emotional stressors can bring about physical pain involves one of my middle-aged male patients who was responding very well to treatment for a chronic lower-back–pain condition. Although he was not supposed to return to my office for a month, he called in for an emergency appointment because of the sudden return of intense pain. When he arrived at my office, the most obvious question to ask was what exactly had happened and when did the pain begin. He stated that he had done no physical activity leading up to the onset of the pain and that he first experienced the pain while seated in a movie theater with his wife.

I performed my usual analysis of his spine, determined which areas needed correction, and proceeded with my chiropractic treatment. My experience, however, told me there was probably more to this than an ergonomically incorrect movie theater seat as the causal factor in his back pain, so I tested him for a neuro-emotional complex.

In this particular case, it turned out that he and his wife had been debating over which movie to see, and although he really did not want to see the one she had chosen, they saw it anyway. So there he was, sitting in the movie theater, grumbling all the way through a movie he had already decided he hated before he even saw it, and the stress caused his back to go into a spasm so that he could barely get up out of his chair by the time the movie was over. Now, at first glance, this would all seem to be a rather immature response over something as silly as a movie, but there's more.

Further testing revealed that this was just the tip of the iceberg and that the origin of this type of emotional response for him was his *wedding*, which had taken place *thirty-eight years* ago! He had wanted a small, intimate wedding with just close family and friends, but his lovely bride-to-be had insisted on a major extravaganza that included nearly every person she had ever known in her life. He conceded and let her have her way, and it had been gnawing at him for all the years since. Now, when a similar contentious situation arose, it literally rang his wedding bells and resulted in an emotional charge that affected his body. By using the neuro-emotional technique, we broke the connection between the emotional response and the corresponding physical reaction. After thirty-eight years of carrying around these emotions, it is probable that similar emotional conflicts will arise, but with this technique, the physical consequences will not reccur.

BEING "RIGHT" CAN BE VERY PAINFUL

An example of one of the most tragic and extreme examples of a neuro-emotional complex as the underlying cause of a pain syndrome involved a forty-two-year-old man who had a work-related lifting injury that resulted in unusually severe back pain. The man was originally employed by a state-of-the-art medical supply company that shipped high-tech surgical tools to hospitals, sometimes on immediate notice to save someone's life. He was in charge of handling the phone orders and getting the shipments out, a job with a lot of control and, in his perception, power.

Unfortunately, as time went on and the company's competitors developed more advanced surgical tools, business slowed down dramatically, and the company was looking to downsize by getting rid of employees with the most seniority and the highest wages. Because the company's employees were unionized, it was not easy to simply fire people without incurring legal difficulties, so they transferred this guy to the shipping department. In his mind, he went from a powerful white-collar job to a guy in overalls doing manual labor.

The actual event that caused his injury was lifting a five-pound box of surgical gloves. It resulted in intense, debilitating lower-back pain that forever changed his life. He was treated by orthopedic specialists, neurologists, and physical therapists. He received cortisone injections in his spine, eventually had two surgeries to try to relieve nerve pressure, and finding little to no resolution for his pain, was placed on lifetime disability. Thus a big lawsuit followed.

When he came to see me ten years after the initial injury, he was still in considerable pain and unable to sit, stand, or walk comfortably. It was obvious from our first consultation that he blamed his former employer for everything that was wrong with his life, and it occurred to me that there was probably a neuro-emotional complex involved in his pain syndrome.

I don't usually start with the neuro-emotional technique on a patient's first visit, but this guy had been through so much other care for his back pain with such minimal results that I thought it was in his best interest to at least explore this avenue. I explained to him that while there was certainly something structurally wrong with his spine, there might also be a chemical or emotional component that was contributing to his pain. He was pretty much willing to try anything at this point, so after examining him and treating him with spinal manipulation, I tested him for a neuro-emotional complex.

In going through the procedure it became apparent that the emotional content underlying his back pain was anger, and it was quite a revelation to him when he realized that it was his bitter anger at being demoted that was actually causing most of his pain. What became clear to him was that, in his mind, he couldn't get well because if he did, he would have to go back to a job that he perceived as humiliating and beneath his qualifications. It was emotionally so painful to go back to that job that it subconsciously transformed into physical pain that made him unable to work. In addition, his physical condition justified, at least in his mind, his blame and hatred of the company, like a bad song that played continuously in his head. This man actually recovered to the point where his pain was so diminished (having two surgeries does tend to permanently alter normal spinal dynamics) that he was able to return to work as a consultant for another company.

The lesson to be learned from this, and it is one that I frequently mention to other patients with similar issues, is that sometimes being "right" can be a very painful experience. Harboring anger, blame, animosity, and resentment in the name of being justified or "right" in one's opinions and beliefs can lead to all kinds of mischief and negative health consequences. To paraphrase a quote from Mother Teresa, no matter how large the hurt or anger is, there comes a time when you simply have to let it go and move on with your life. This patient had wasted years of his life being angry and in pain, when in the end, he ended up doing what he should have done in the first place, which was to leave a job he no longer liked and transfer his talent and expertise to a new employer.

These are cases of patients whose pain syndromes were not resolved by using physical modalities (chiropractic manipulation, physical therapy, massage, surgery) or hormonal/nutritional balancing, because the driving force behind their pain had an emotional component. This is not to imply that every person with a pain syndrome has an emotional basis for it, or that if there is one, it has to be due to some severe emotional trauma. Sometimes a persistent pain in the neck is nothing more emotionally charged than having a coworker who is particularly irritating. But if seeing that person five days a week is the cause of your pain, then the neuro-emotional technique is an excellent way to resolve it.

It is very important to note that neuro-emotional technique does not, nor has it ever been intended to, replace psychiatric care or psychological counseling. It certainly can be a helpful adjunct in cases where a patient has received such care, and in so doing, has come to an intellectual understanding of his problems but continues to respond negatively to the same old triggers. In such cases neuro-emotional technique can be enormously beneficial.

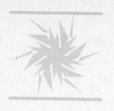

CONCLUSION

We have come full circle in exploring all of the components of stress and how to cope with each one of them. Hopefully, you are now able to see stress in a very different light and to realize that it may not be your external circumstances alone that are causing you to feel stressed-out; that in many instances, it has more to do with your internal structural, chemical, and emotional well-being. Whether it requires seeking appropriate treatment to relieve pain and eliminate the need for NSAIDs, repairing intestinal-tract damage and resolving inflammation, measuring and correcting cortisol imbalances, choosing to eat properly, and/or learning to truly understand what your opinions and judgments are and how deeply they affect your life, you can regain your health and have a blueprint for managing stress successfully.

When I first decided to write this book, my purpose was to be able to take the procedures I do successfully on a daily basis in my practice and extend them to a larger audience. While it is enormously fulfilling to help people regain their health on an individual basis, it became increasingly apparent, and alarming, that there are millions of people suffering from the effects of cortisol imbalances. As we have seen, these people have no idea that intestinal-tract and/or systemic inflammation can be the cause of their feeling so stressed-out, nor are they aware of the many symptoms that can result from cortisol imbalance. At its most tragic endpoint, the symptoms of cortisol imbalance erodes health and ruins lives.

From a clinical perspective, if there are only two things that writing this book accomplishes, I want them to be: (1) that doctors include salivary cortisol testing as a routine part of a complete physical exam and (2) that everyone who is prescribed or is taking NSAIDs is also taking L-glutamine, so that 103,000 people won't be hospitalized and 16,500 people will no longer die each year from gastric bleeding. I want the fact that L-glutamine prevents the negative side effects of NSAIDs to become so well known that doctors who fail to prescribe L-glutamine for their patients when they prescribe NSAIDs will be considered guilty of malpractice if the patient ends up in the hospital or dies from intestinal bleeding. In ten years, 165,000 lives could be saved.

It is my sincere hope that you will use any or all of the resources listed at the end of this book to help you find out what your cortisol levels are, and how to resolve any imbalances that might be present in your triangle of health.

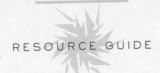

LABORATORIES FOR HORMONE TESTING

Diagnos-Techs, Inc.

6620 192nd Place, Bldg. J
Kent, WA 98032
425-251-0596
e-mail: cs@diagnostechs.com

Great Smokies Diagnostic Laboratory

63 Zillicon Street
Asheville, NC 28801
800-522-4762

Meridian Valley Laboratory

515 West Harrison Street, Suite 9
Kent, WA 98032
253-859-8700

CHIROPRACTIC CARE AND SPECIFIC ADJUSTING TECHNIQUES

American Chiropractic Association

1701 Claredon Blvd.
Arlington, VA 22209
800–986–4636

International Chiropractic Association

1110 N. Glebe Road, Suite 1000
Arlington, VA 22201
800–423–4690

Activator Methods: This chiropractic adjusting technique uses a handheld adjusting instrument that delivers a specific, light thrust to the joint being treated. It is very gentle, and there is no cracking or popping of the joints. To find a chiropractor near you who uses this method, call 800-598-0224.

Direct Non-Force Technique (DNFT): This method is also very gentle and adjusts the joints by using a quick thrust of the doctor's thumb on the joint being treated. To find a chiropractor near you who uses this technique, call 213-657-2338.

Sacro-Occipital Technique: This technique uses cushioned wedges specifically placed under the patient, allowing gravity to realign the lower back. The technique also adjusts joints in the more traditional manner of applying a quick thrust to the joints that causes a popping sound, and includes cranial adjusting. To find a chiropractor who uses this method, check the website www.sorsi.com or search the Internet for Chiropractic + Sacro Occipital Technique.

NUTRITIONAL SUPPLEMENTS

D.S.D. International, Ltd.: Distributor of Biotics nutritional supplements in California, Arizona, and New Mexico. To find a doctor who is familiar with these supplements, call 800-232-3183.

Biotics Research Corporation: The manufacturer of Biotics nutritional supplements; call 800-231-5777.

Apex Energetics

800-736-4381

Website

Visit my website at www.richardweinsteindc.com for updated information regarding cortisol and hormone research and continuing new strategies for regaining and maintaining vibrant health.

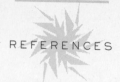
CHAPTER 4. TESTING CORTISOL LEVELS

Baxendale, P. M.; and James, V. H. T. 1983. *Immunoassays for Clinical Chemistry.* New York: Churchill Livingstone, 430–44.

Berthonneau, J.; Tanguy, G.; Janssens, Y.; et al. 1989. *Human Reprod.* 4: 625–28.

Connor, M. L.; Sanford, L. M.; and Howland, B. E. 1982. *Can. J. Physiol. Pharmacol.* 60: 410–13.

Cook, N. J.; Read, G. F.; Walker, R. F.; Harris, B.; and Riad-Fahmy, D. 1986. *Eur. J. Appl. Physiol.* 55: 634–38.

DeBoever, J.; Kohen, F.; Bouve, J.; Leyseele, D.; and Vanderkerckhove, D. 1990. *Clin. Chem.* 36: 2036–41.

Evans, J. J.; Stewart, C. R.; and Merrick, A. Y. 1980. *Br. J. Obstet. Gynaecol.* 87: 624–26.

Ferguson, D. B. 1984. *Front. Oral Physiol.* 5: 1–162.

Fischer-Rasmussen, W.; Gabrielsen, M. V.; and Wisborg, T. 1982. *Acta. Obstet. Gynecol.* 60: 417–20.

Frisch, R. E. 1987. *Hum. Reprod.* 2: 521–33.

Gaskell, S. J.; Pike, A. W.; and Griffiths, K. 1980. *Steroids.* 36: 219–28.

Gould, V. J.; Turkes, A. O.; and Gaskell, S. J. 1986. *J. Steroid Biochem.* 24: 563–67.

Guechot, J., et al. 1987. *Neuropsychobiology.* 18: 1–4.

Kahn, J. P.; Rubinow, D. R.; Davis, C. L.; Kling, M.; and Post, R. M. 1988. *Biol. Psychiatry.* 23: 335–49.

Laudat, M. H.; Cerdas, S.; Fourier, C.; and Guiban, D.; et al. 1988. *J. Clin. Endocrinol. Metab.* 66: 343–48.

Lipson, S. F., and Ellison, P. T. 1989. *Am. J. Human Biol.* 1: 249–55.

Malamud, D. 1992. *Br. Med. J.* 305: 207–8.

Mandel, I. D. 1993. *Ann. N.Y. Acad. Sci.* 694: 1–10.

Mandel, I. D. 1990 *Oral Pathol.* 19: 119–25.

Meulenberg, P. M., and Hoffman, J. A. 1989. *Clin. Chem.* 35: 168–72.

Mounib, N.; Sultan, C. H.; Bringer, J.; Hedon, B.; Nicolas, J. C.; Cristol, P.; Bressot, N.; and Descomps. 1988. *J. Steroid Biochem.* 31: 861–65.

O'Connor, P.; and Corrigan, D. L. 1987. *Med. Sci. Sports Exercise.* 19: 224–28.

Peters, L. R.; Walker, R. F.; Riad-Fahmy, D.; and Hall, R. 1982. *Clin. Endocrinol.* 17: 583–92.

Ratcliffe, J. G. 1985. *Adrenal Cortex.* Eds. Anderson, D. C., and Winter, J. D. 188–205.

Read, G. F.; Harper, M. E.; Peeling, W. B.; and Griffiths, K. 1981. *Int. J. Androl.* 4: 623–27.

Robinson, J.; Walker, S.; Read, G. F.; and Riad-Fahmy, D. 1981. *Lancet.* 1111–12.

Smith, R. G.; Besch, P. K.; Dill, B.; and Buttram Jr., V. C. 1979. *Fertil. Steril.* 31: 513.

Tarui, H., and Nakamura, A. 1987. *Aviat. Space Environ. Med.* 58: 573–75.

Tunn, S.; Mollmann, H.; Barth, J.; Derendorf, H.; and Kreig, M. 1992. *Clin. Chem.* 38: 1491–94.

Turkes, A. O., and Read, G. F. 1984. *Immunoassays of Steroids in Saliva.* Cardiff: Alpha Omega, 228–38.

Umeda, T.; Hiramatsu, R.; Iwaoka, T.; Shimada, T.; Miura, F.; and Sato, T. 1981. *Clin. Chem. Acta.* 110: 245–53.

Vining, R. F.; McGinley, R. A.; Maksvytis, J. J.; and Ho, K. Y. 1983. *Ann. Clin. Biochem.* 20: 329–35.

Vining, R. F.; McGinley, R. A.; and Symons, R. G. 1983. *Clin. Chem.* 29: 1752–56.

Vuorento, T.; Lahti, A.; Hovatta, O.; Huhtaniemi, I., 1989. *Scand. J. Clin. Lab. Invest.* 49: 395–401.

Walker, R., et al. 1982. Ninth Tenovus Workshop, Cardiff, U.K.

Walker, R. F.; Wilson, D. W.; Read, G. F.; and Riad-Fahmy, D. 1980. *Int. J. Androl.* 3: 105.

Walker, S. M.; Walker, R. F.; and Riad-Fahmy, D. 1984. *Horm. Res.* 20: 231–40.

Wong, Y. F.; Mao, K.; Panesar, N.; Loong, E. P. L.; Chang, A. M. Z.; and Mi, Z. J. 1990. *Eur. J. Obstet. Gynecol. Reprod. Biol.* 34: 129–35.

CHAPTER 5. THE RELATIONSHIP OF CORTISOL TO OTHER DISEASES

Almy, T., 1951. "Experimental studies on irritable colon," *Amer. J. Med.* 10: 60.

Barnes, B. O., and Galton, L. 1976. *Hypothyroidism: the Unsuspected Illness.* New York: Harper & Row.

Bird, C. E.; Masters, V.; and Clark, A. F. 1984. "Dehydroepiandrosterone sulfate: kinetics of metabolism in normal young men and women," *Clin. Invest. Med.* 7: 119–22.

Born, J., et al. 1991. "Gluco- and antimineralocorticoid effects on human sleep: a role of central corticosteroid receptors," *Amer. J. Physiol.* E183–E188.

Born, J., et al. 1986. "Night-time plasma cortisol secretion is associated with specific sleep stages," *Bio. Psychiat.* 21: 1415–24.

Buske-Kirschbaum, A.; Jobst, S.; Psych, D.; Wustmans, A.; Kirschbaum, C.; Rauh, W.; and Hellhammer, D. 1997. "Cortisol responses to psychosocial stress in children with atopic disorders," *Psychosomatic Med.*

Carroll, B. J., et al. 1981. "A specific laboratory for the diagnosis of melancholia," *Arch. Gen. Psychiat.* 38: 15–22.

Carroll, B. J., et al. 1976. "Neuroendocrine regulation in depression," *Arch. Gen. Psychiat.* 33: 1051–58.

Champe, P. C., and Harvey, R. A. 1992. *Lippinncott Illustrated Reviews.* Biochemistry.

Cleary, M. P., and Zisk, J. F. 1986. "Anti-obesity effect of two different levels of dehydroepiandrosterone in lean and obese middle-aged female zucker rats," *Int. J. Obesity.* 10: 193–204.

Croes, M. P., et al. 1993. "Cortisol reaction in success and failure condition in endogenous depressed patients and controls," *Psychoneuroendocrin.* 18: 23–35.

Cutolo, M.; Balleari, E.; Giusti, M.; et al. 1991. "Androgen replacement therapy in male patients with rheumatoid arthritis," *Arthritis Rheum.* 34: 1–5.

De Feo, P., et al. 1989. "Contribution of cortisol to glucose counterregulation in humans," *Amer. J. Physiol.* 257: E35–E42.

Demitrack, M. A., et al. 1991. "Evidence for impaired activation of the hypothalamic-pituitary-adrenal axis in patients with chronic fatigue syndrome," *J. Clin. Endocrin. Metab.* 73: 1224–34.

Desiderado, O.; MacKinnon, J.; and Hissom, R. 1974. "Development of gastric ulcers following stress termination," *J. Comp. and Physiol. Psych.* 87: 208.

Dey, A. C., et al. 1972. "Excretion of conjugated 11-deoxy-17-ketosteriods in 'Essential' hypertension," *Can. J. Biochem.* 50: 1273–81.

Donald, R. A., et al. 1994. Plasma corticotrophin releasing hormone, vasopressin, ACTH and cortisol responses to acute myocardial infarction," *Clin. Endocrin.* 40: 499–504.

Feldman, M.; Walker, P.; Green, J.; and Weingarden, K. 1986. "Life events, stress and psychosocial factors in men with peptic ulcer disease: a multidimensional case-controlled study," *Gastroenterol.* 91: 1370.

Foldes, J., et al. 1983. "Dehydroepiandrosterone sulfate (DS), dehydroepiandrosterone (D), and 'free' dehydroepiandrosterone (FD) in the plasma with thyroid diseases," *Horm. Metab. Res.* 15: 623–24.

Freiss, E.; Trachsel, L.; Guldner, J.; Schier, T.; Steiger, A.; and Holsboer, F. 1995. "DHEA administration increases rapid eye movement sleep and EEG power in the sigma frequency range," *Am. J. of Physiol.* 268 (Endorcrin Metab. 31): E107–E113.

Gansler, T.; Meller, S.; and Cleary, J., 1985. "Chronic administration of dehydroepiandrosterone reduces pancreatic B-cell hyperplasia and hyperinsulinemia in genetically obese zucker rats," *Proc. Soc. Exp. Biol. Med.* 180: 155–62.

Gheorghiu, T., and Hubner, G. 1975. "Morphological and functional gastric changes in stress ulcer," *Experimental Ulcer: Models, Methods, and Clinical Validity*. Baden–Baden: Witzstrock.

Hall, G. M.; Perry, L. A.; and Spector, T. D. 1993. "Depressed levels of dehydroepiandrosterone sulfate in postmenstrual women with rheumatoid arthritis but no relation with axial bone density," *Am. Rheum.* 52: 211–14.

Hedman, M.; Nilsson, E.; and de la Torre, B. 1989. "Low sulpho-conjugated steroid hormone levels in systemic lupus erythematosus," *Clin. Exp. Rheumatol.* 7: 583–88.

Heimke, C., et al, 1994. "Circadian variations in antigen-specific proliferation of human T lymphocytes and correlation to cortisol production," *Psychoneoroendocrin.* 20: 335–42.

Holmes, G. P., et al. 1987. "A cluster of patients with a chronic mononucleosis-like syndrome: Is Epstein-Barr virus the cause? *JAMA.* 257: 2297–2302.

Hong Din, J. U., et al. 1988. "High serum cortisol levels in exercise associated amenorrhea," *Ann. Int. Med.* 108: 530–34.

Kaplan, J. "Social behavior and gender in biomedical investigations using monkeys: Studies in atherogenesis," *Laboratory Animal Science.*

Kumar, D., and Wingate, D. 1988. "Irritable bowel syndrome," *An Illustrated Guide to Gastrointestinal Motility.* Chichester: John Wiley.

Manolagas, S. C., et al. 1979. "Adrenal steroids and the development of osteoporosis in the oophorectomized women," *Lancet.* 2: 597.

Marin, P., et al. 1992. "Cortisol secretion in relation to body fat distribution in obese menopausal women," *Metab.* 41: 882–86.

Meikle, A. W., et al. 1992. "The presence of dehydroepiandrosterone-specific receptor binding complex in murine T cells," *Am. J. Med Sci.* 303: 366–71.

Miller, J. E., et al. 1994. "Characterization of 24 hour cortisol release in obese and non-obese hyperandrogenic women," *Gynecol. Endocrin.* 8: 247–54.

Murison, R., and Bakke, H. 1990. "The role of corticotrophin-releasing factor in rat gastric ulcerogenesis," *Neurobiology of Stress Ulcers.* Annals of the New York Academy of Sciences, vol. 597.

Nordin, B. E. C., et al. 1985. "The relation between calcium absorption, serum dehydroepiandrosterone, and vertebral mineral density in postmenopausal women," *J. Clinic. Endocrin. Metab.* 60: 651–57.

Nowaczynski, W., et al. 1967. "Further evidence of altered adrenocortical function in hypertension. Dehydroepiandrosterone excretion rate," *Can. J. Biochem.* 46: 1031–38.

Opstad, K. 1994. "Circadian rhythm of hormones is extinguished during prolonged physical stress, sleep and energy deficiency in young men," *Eur. J. Endocrin.* 131: 56–66.

Reaven, G.; Bernstein, R.; Davis, B.; and Olefski, J. 1976. "Nonketotic diabetes mellitus: Insulin deficiency or insulin resistance?" *Amer. J. Med.*

Sachar, E. J., et al. 1973. "Disrupted 24 hour patterns of cortisol secretion in depressive illness," *Arch. Gen. Psychiat.* 28: 19–24.

Schuster, M. 1989. "Mucus secretion decreases with stress and glucocorticoid administration." In Sleisenger, M., and Fordtron, J. *Gastrointestinal Disease: Pathophysiology, Diagnosis, Management,* 4th ed. Philadelphia: Saunders.

Stahl, H., et al. 1992. "Dehydroepiandrosterone levels in patients with prostatic cancer, heart diseases, and under surgery stress," *Exp. Clin. Endocrin.* 99: 68–70.

Straus, S., et al. 1998. *J. Allergy and Clin. Immunol.* 81: 79.

Suzuki, T.; Suzuki, N.; Engleman, E. G.; Mizushima, Y.; and Sakane, T. 1995. "Low serum levels of dehydroepiandrosterone may cause deficient IL-2 production by lymphocytes in patients with systemic lupus erythematosus," *Clin. Exp. Immunol.* 99: 251–55.

Thompson, D.; Richelson, E.; and Malagelada, J. 1982. "Perturbation of gastric emptying and duodenal motility through the central nervous system," *Gastroenterol.* 83: 1200.

Von Zerssen, D., et al. 1987. "Diurnal variation of mood and the cortisol rhythm in depression and normal states of mind," *Eur. Arch. Psychiat. Neurol. Sci.* 237: 36–45.

Williams, Janice, *Circulation.* Chapel Hill: University of North Carolina.

CHAPTER 6. RESOLVING CORTISOL IMBALANCES

Akgul, A., and Kivane, M. 1988. "Inhibitory effects of selected Turkish spices and oregano components on some food-borne fungi," *Int. J. Food Microbiology.* 6: 263.

Alverdy, J. A. 1990. "The effect of total parenteral nutrition in gut lamina propria cells," *J. Parent Enteral. Nutr.* 14 (suppl.).

Conner, D. E., and Beuchat, L. D. 1984. "Effects of essential oils from plants on growth of food spoilage yeasts," *J. Food Science.* 49: 429.

Deighton, N.; Glidewell, S. M.; Deans, S. G.; and Goodman, B. A. 1933.

"Identification by EPR spectroscopy of carvacrol and thymol as the major sources of free radicals in the oxidation of plant essential oils," *J. Science Food Agriculture.* 63: 221.

Fox, A. D., et al. 1988. "Effects of glutamine-supplemented enteral diet on methotrexate-induced enterocolitis," *JPEN.* 12: 325–31.

Fuert, S., and Fox, L. "Effects of orally administrating Spanish moss," *Science.* 1053: 626–27.

Gardner, M. L. G. 1988. "Gastrointestinal absorption of intact proteins," *Annu. Rev. Nutrition.* 8: 329–50.

Gardner, M. L. G. 1984. "Intestinal assimilation of intact peptides and proteins from the diet, a neglected field," *Biol. Rev.* 59: 289–331.

Genova, R., and Guerra, A. 1988. "A thymomodulin management of food allergy," *Int. J. Tiss. React.* 8: 239–42.

Gibson, G. R., et al. 1995. "Dietary modification of the human microbiota: introducing the concept of prebiotics," *J. Nutrition.* 125: 1401–12.

Haigler, E. D. 1972. "Response to orally administered synthetic thyrotropin-releasing hormone in man," *J. Clin. Endocrinol. Metab.* 631–35.

Hidaka, H., et al. 1990. "The effects of undigestible fructooligosaccharides on intestinal microflora and various physiological functions on human health," *New Developments in Dietary Fiber.* New York: Plenum Press. 105–117.

Huang, K. F. 1983. "Study of the absorption of peptide from thymus extract when administered orally," *Erfahrungs-Heilkunde.* Bd32, H. 11.

Iantomai, T., et al. 1994. "Glutathione metabolism in Crohn's disease," *Biochem. Med. Metab. Biol.* 53: 87–91.

Julius, M., et al. 1994. "Glutathione and morbidity in a community-based sample of elderly," *J. Clin. Epidemiol.* 47: 1021–26.

Kumar, U. 1996. "Purification and characterization of chromogranin-A from the adrenal glands of human and bovine donors," *Biochem. Mol. Biol. Int.* 40: 83–91.

Lin, C-Y., and Low, T. L. K. 1989. "A comparative study of the immunological effects of bovine and porcine thymic extracts: induction of lymphoproliferative responses and enhancement of interleukin-2, interferon and tumor necrotic factor production in vitro on cord blood lymphocytes," *Immuno. Pharmacol.* 18: 1–10.

Lin, C-Y., et al. 1987. "Treatment of combined immunodeficiency with thymic extract," *Annals. Allergy.* 58: 379–84.

Miller, J. M., and Ophershaw. 1964. "The increased proteolytic activity of human blood serum after the oral administration of bromelain," *Exp. Med. Surg.* 22: 277–80.

Monteleone, P.; Maj, M.; Beinat, L.; Natale, M.; and Kemali, D. 1992. "Blunting by chronic phosphatidylserine administration of the stress-induced activation of the hypothalamo–pituitary–adrenal axis in healthy men," *European J. Clin. Pharmacol.* 42(4): 385–88.

Monteleone, P.; Maj, M.; Beinat, L.; Tanzillo, C.; and Kemali, D. 1990. "Effects of phosphatidylserine on the neuroendocrine response to physical stress in humans," *Neuroendocrinol.* 52(3): 243–58.

Morton, J. F. *Atlas of Medicinal Plants of Middle America.* Springfield, Ill.: Charles C. Thomas.

Murch, S. H., et al. 1993. "Disruption of sulfated glycosaminoglycan in intestinal inflammation," *Lancet.* 341: 711–14.

Okabe, S.; Takeuchi, K.; Honda, K.; and Takagi, K. 1976. "Effects of acetylsalicylic acid (ASA), ASA plus L-glutamine and L-glutamine on healing of chronic gastric ulcer in the rat," *Digestion.* 14: 85–88.

Oota, K., et al. 1976. "Clinical studies of Hi-Z pills on indefinite complaints of gastrointestinal neurosis, Yakuri to Chiryo," 4: 113.

Sezik, E.; Tumen, G.; et al. 1933. "Essential oil composition of four *origanum vulgare* subspecies of Anatolian origin," *J. Essent. Oil Res.* 5: 425–31.

Souba, W. W.; Smith, R. J.; and Wilmore, D. W. 1985. "Glutamine metabolism by the intestinal tract," *JPEN* 9: 608–17.

Steffen, C., et al. 1979. "Untersuchungen über intestinale Resorption mit 3H-markiertem, Enzymgemisch," *Acta. Med. Aust.* 6: 13–18.

Stein, J. 1967. "Objective demonstration of the organ-specific effectiveness of cellular preparations." In Schmidt, F., ed. *Cell Research and Cellular Therapy.* Ott Publishers. 294–301.

Svensen, A. B.; and Scheffer, J. J. C. 1985. *Essential Oils and Aromatic Plants.* Martinus Nijoff/W. Junk Publishers.

Vidaly Plama, R. R., et al. 1978. "Articular cartilage pharmacology: In vitro studies of glucosamine and nonsteroidal inflammatory drugs," *Pharm. Res. Commun.* 10: 557–69.

Wilmore, W. D. 1992. "The effect of glutamine on the gastrointestinal tract," *Rivista Ital. di Nutriz. Parent ed Enter.* 10: 1–6.

Wilson, J. L. 1996. "The anti-aging effects of liquid thymus extracts." In Klatz, R. ed. *Advances in Anti-Aging Medicine.* Vol. 1, 349–55.

Windmueller, H. G. 1982. "Glutamine Utilization by the Small Intestine," *Adv. Enzymol.* 53. 201–37.

Winslet, M. C., et al. 1994. "Mucosal glucosamine synthetase activity in inflammatory bowel disease," *Dig. Disease Sci.* 39: 540–44.

Yagi, Ohishi. 1976. "Action of ferulic acid and its derivatives as antioxidants," *J. Nutri. Sci. Vitaminol.* 206: 127.

Yokahama, S. 1984. "Intestinal absorption mechanisms of thyrotropin-releasing hormone," *J. Pharm. Dyn.* 7: 445–51.

Yoshimura, K., et al. 1993. "Effect of enteral glutamine administration on experimental inflammatory bowel disease," *JPEN.* 17: 235.

Zaloga, G. P. 1994. *Nutrition in Critical Care.* Mosby. 552–53.

CHAPTER 7. MAKE THE PAIN GO AWAY

Dean, D. H., and Schmidt, R. M. 1992. "A comparison of the costs of chiropractors versus alternative medical practitioners." Richmond, Virginia: University of Richmond.

Demographic Characteristics of Users of Chiropractic Services. 1991. The Gallup Organization. Princeton, New Jersey.

Ebrall, P. S. June 1992. "Mechanical low-back pain: a comparison of medical and chiropractic management within the Victorian work care scheme," *Chiropractic J. Australia.* 22 (2): 47–53.

Evidence Report: Behavioral and Physical Treatments for Tension-Type and Cervicogenic Headaches. May 2000. Duke University, Evidence-based Practice Center.

Hayek, Ray. 2002. *Advance.* 23: 2, 4.

Jarvis, K. B.; Phillips, R. B.; et al. August 1991. "Cost per case comparison of back injury claims of chiropractic versus medical management for conditions with identical diagnostic codes," *J. Occupational Med.* 33 (8): 847–52.

Kandel, Eric. 2000. *Principles of Neural Science.* 482–85.

Ketsroser, D. B. February 2002. *Minnesota Medicine.* 83: 51–54.

Koes, B. W.; Bouter, L. M.; et al. 1992. "Randomized clinical trial of manipulative therapy and physiotherapy for persistent back and neck complaints: results of one year follow up," *Brit. Med. J.* 304: 601–5.

MacDonald, M. J., and Morton, L. January 1986. "Chiropractic evaluation study task III report of the relevant literature," MRI Project No. 8533-D, for Department of Defense. OCHAMPUS. Aurora, Colorado.

Mayer, D.; Price, D.; Barber, J.; and Rafi, A. 1976. "Acupuncture analgesia: evidence for activation of a pain inhibitory system as a mechanism of action," *Advances in Pain Research and Therapy.* 1: 751.

Meade, T. W.; Dyer, S., et al. 1990. "Low back pain of mechanical origin: randomized comparison of chiropractic and hospital outpatient treatment," *Brit. Med. J.* 300 (67137): 1431–37.

Shekelle, P. G.; Adams, A.; et al. 1992. "The appropriateness of spinal manipulation for lower-back pain," Santa Monica, Calif.: RAND Corporation.

Steward, Oswald. 2000. *Functional Neuroscienc.* New York: Springer. 218–19.

Wiberg, J. M. N.; Nordsteen, J.; and Nilsson, N. 1988. "The short-term effect of spinal manipulation in the treatment of infantile colic: a randomized controlled trial with a blinder observer," *J. Manip. Physiol. Ther.* 199: 22(8): 517–22; Klougart, N.; Nilsson, N.; and Jacobsen, J. 1989. "Infantile colic treated by chiropractors: a prospective study of 316 cases," *J. Manip. Physiol. Ther.* 12: 281–88; Lucassen, P. L.; Assendelft, W. J.; et al. 1988. "Effectiveness of treatments for infantile colic: systemic review" (published erratum appears in *BMJ.* 31 [7152]:171), *BMJ.* 316(7144): 1563–69; Adams, L. M., and Davidson, M. 1997. "Present concepts of infantile colic," *Pediatr. Ann.* 16: 817–20; Hide, D. W., and Guyer, B. M. 1983. "Prevalence of infantile colic," *Arch. Dis. Child.* 57(7): 559–60.

Wolk, S. September 1988. "Chiropractic versus medical care: a cost analysis of disability and treatment for back-related workers' compensation cases," Arlington, Virginia: Foundation for Chiropractic Education and Research.

Woodward, M. J.; Cook, et al. 1996. "Chiropractic treatment of chronic whiplash," *Injury.* 27(9): 643–45.

Chapter 8. The Not-So-Common Commonsense Diet

Barberger-Gateau, P.; Letenneur, L.; Deschamps, V.; Peres, K.; Dartigues, J-F.; and Renaud, S. October 26, 2002. "Fish, meat, and risk of dementia: a cohort study," *Brit. Med. J.* 325: 932–33.

Hu, F. B., and Willet, W. C. November 27, 2002. "Optimal diets for prevention of coronary disease," *JAMA*. 288: 2569–78.

Miyamoto, H.; Saura, R.; Doita, M.; Kurasaka, M.; and Mizuno, K. November 15, 2002. "The role of cyclooxygenase-2 in lumbar disc herniation," *Spine*. 27(22): 2477–83.

Murray, M. July/August 1995. "GLA vs. omega-3 fatty acids in rheumatoid arthritis," *Amer. J. Nat. Med*. 2: 9–11.

Peet, M.; Glen, I.; and Horrobin, D. 2000. *Phospholipid Spectrum Disorder in Psychiarty*. Marius Press.

San Jose Mercury News. January 11, 2003, p. 2.

Schlosser, E. 2000. *Fast Food Nation*. Boston: Houghton Mifflin.

CHAPTER 10. THE EMOTIONAL COMPONENT OF ILLNESS

Basmajian, J. V. 1989. *Biofeedback, Principals and Practice for Clinicians*. 3rd. ed. Baltimore, MD: Williams & Wilkins.

Bohannon, R. 1997. "Internal consistency of manual muscle testing scores," *Perceptual and Motor Skills*. 85: 736–38.

Bohannon, R. 1997. "Reference values for extremity muscle strength obtained by hand-held dynamometry from adults ages 20 to 70," *Arch. Phys. Med. and Rehab*. 78: 26–32.

Bonnet, M.; Bradley, M. M.; Lang, P. J.; and Requin, J. 1995. "Modulation of spinal reflexes; arousal, pleasure, and action," *Psychophysiol*. 32: 367–72.

Bradley, M. M.; Cuthbert, B. N.; and Lang, P. J. 1996. "Picture media and emotions: effects of a sustained affective context," *Psychophysiol*. 33: 662–70.

Bradley, M. T., and Cullen, M. C. 1993. "Polygraph lie detection on real events in a laboratory setting," *Perceptual and Motor Skills*. 76: 1051–58.

Burton, D. 1988. "Do anxious swimmers swim slower? Reexamining the elusive anxiety-performance relationship," *J. Sport and Exercise Psych*. 10: 45–61.

Cacioppo, J. T.; Uchino, B. N.; Crites, S. L.; Snydersmith, M. A.; Smith, G.; Bernstein, G. G.; and Lang, P. J. 1992. "Relationship between facial expressiveness and sympathetic activation in emotion: a critical review, with emphasis on modeling underlying mechanisms and individual differences," *J. Personality and Social Psych*. 62: 110–128.

Coren, S. 1993. "Measurement of handedness via self-report: the relationship between brief and extended inventories," *Perceptual and Motor Skills*. 76: 1035–42.

De Melo, F., and Laurent, M. 1996. "Effects of competitive activation on precision movement control," *Perceptual and Motor Skills*. 83: 1203–8.

Fischler, I.; Achariyapaopan, T.; and Perry, N. W. 1985. "Brain potentials during sentence verification: automatic aspects of comprehension," *Biol. Psych*. 23: 81–106.

Goodheart, G. 1964. *Applied Kinesiology*. Detroit, MI: private printing.

Gould, D.; Jackson, S.; and Finch, L. 1993. "Sources of stress in national figure skaters," *J. Sport and Exercise Physiol*. 15: 134–59.

Hsieh, C-Y., and Phillips, R. B. 1990. "Reliability of manual muscle testing with a computerized dynamometer," *J. Manip. and Physiol. Therapeutics*. 13: 72–82.

Lawson, A., and Calderon, L. 1997. "Interexaminer agreement for applied kinesiology manual muscle testing," *Perceptual and Motor Skill*. 84: 539–46.

Leisman, G.; Aenhausern, R.; Ferentz, A.; Terfer, T.; and Zemcov, A. 1995. "Electromyographic effects of fatigue and task repetition on the validity of strong and weak muscle estimates in Applied Kinesiological muscle testing," *Perceptual and Motor Skills*. 80: 933–46.

Levinson, R. W.; Ekman, P.; and Friesen, V. W. 1990. "Voluntary facial action emotion-specific autonomic nervous system activity," *Psychophysiol*. 27: 363–84.

Pennebaker, J. W.; Hughes, C. F.; and O'Heeron, R. C. 1987. "The psychophysiology of confession: linking inhibitory and psychosomatic processes," *J. Personality and Social Psych*. 52: 781–93.

Peterson, K. B. 1997. "The effects of spinal manipulation on the intensity of emotional arousal in phobic subjects exposed to threat stimulus: a randomized, controlled, double-blind clinical trial," *J. Manip. and Physiol. Therapeutics*. 20: 602–6.

Walker, S. 1992. "Ivan Pavlov, his dog, and chiropractic," *The Digest of Chiropractic Economics*. 34: 36–46.

Walker, S. 1996. *Neuro Emotional Technique: N.E.T. Basic Manual*. Encinitas, Calif. N.E.T. Inc.

Walther, D. S. 1990. *Applied Kinesiology, Vol. I: Basic procedures and muscle testing*. Pueblo, Colo.: Systems, D.C.

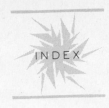

INDEX

E

F

Dr. Richard A. Weinstein has helped hundreds of patients with adrenal-gland and other hormone imbalances, intestinal-tract inflammation, leaky-gut syndrome, Candida infections, and a host of other health disorders. As a chiropractor, he has been in private practice in Capitola, California, for twenty-five years. A 1976 graduate of the New York Chiropractic College, he is a member of: The American Chiropractic Association and its Council on Nutrition, The National Institute of Chiropractic Research, The Foundation for Chiropractic Education and Research, and The California Chiropractic Association. In 1995 and 1996, Dr. Weinstein received the Botterman Award from the California Chiropractic Association for outstanding and dedicated service on behalf of the chiropractic profession.